PRAISE FOR
YOU CAN'T SCREW THIS UP

"In addition to being one of the smartest people in nutrition I've met, [Adam Bornstein is] the perfect person to blaze a better path that provides a more direct, realistic, and effective way to improve your health and mindset and achieve your goals. . . . Consider this your guide to turning that dream into a reality. If you embrace the lessons of *You Can't Screw This Up*, you'll build a more positive mindset and develop healthier habits. And that is the most powerful combination in the world."

—Arnold Schwarzenegger, from the foreword

"It's rare to find someone who makes you believe you can finally eat healthier without all the usual rules and frustrations. Adam is that guy."

—Mike Mancias, NBA athletic trainer, Los Angeles Lakers

"Adam Bornstein is uniquely talented at seeing what the rest of us were staring at but somehow missed. *You Can't Screw This Up* delivers an easy-to-read guide for getting a grip on your relationship with food. It's a wonderful blend of science, experience, and practicality layered on top of his beloved writing style."

—Dr. Andy Galpin, professor and scientist of human performance

"Healthy living can feel like a game where you always lose. This book shows you how to win."

—Michael Easter, author of *The Comfort Crisis*

"The only thing better than Adam's ability to simplify nutrition and psychology into a practical plan is his sincere heart-and-soul desire to make sure you succeed once and for all."

—Jen Widerstrom, former trainer on *The Biggest Loser*

YOU
CAN'T
SCREW
THIS UP

YOU CAN'T SCREW THIS UP

Why Eating Takeout, Enjoying Dessert,
and Taking the Stress Out of Dieting
Leads to Weight Loss That Lasts

ADAM BORNSTEIN

wm

WILLIAM MORROW

An Imprint of HarperCollinsPublishers

HarperCollins books may be purchased for educational, business, or sales promotional use. For information, please email the Special Markets Department at SPsales@harpercollins.com.

A hardcover edition of this book was published in 2023 by William Morrow, an imprint of HarperCollins Publishers.

FIRST WILLIAM MORROW PAPERBACK EDITION PUBLISHED 2024.

Designed by Bonni Leon-Berman
Illustrations by Kiki Garthwaite

Library of Congress Cataloging-in-Publication Data has been applied for.

ISBN 978-0-06-323058-3

24 25 26 27 28 LBC 5 4 3 2 1

DAD,

You were given a death sentence and
turned it into a life sentence. That's the
power of a different mindset. Thanks for
showing me the way. I love you.

CONTENTS

FOREWORD

THERE'S SOMETHING I'VE NEVER understood about the diet industry. It's not discussed very often, but it's a big reason so many people don't see the results they want.

The industry is too damn negative, and the plans you're given are too damn complicated.

Consider this my word of caution: that combination is doing far more harm than you realize, and walking away from it can be one of the healthiest decisions you make.

I'm not sure when it changed, but it's frustrating to see so many plans built around fear and negative motivation. When I look at the amount of shame and guilt, I'm not surprised that so many people have struggled to eat better and exercise consistently. As I sit and watch many people struggle to become healthier, I'm frustrated for them because I see many people who want to change and are motivated to do so.

No one has ever changed by beating themselves up. Change only comes from a positive vision. Being negative about how you look won't move you closer to health; having a positive vision of how healthy you want to be is the only path forward.

As if that wasn't bad enough, once they make you feel awful about yourself with paralyzing negativity, they make you feel like you need a Ph.D. to know how to eat. They change the trends once a month and invent new words for every new fad.

If I've learned anything after more than sixty years of promoting better health, you have to build up the mind just as much as the body if you want to achieve your goals. And once you have a vision of where you want to be, it can happen with small steps. Taking a walk or doing bodyweight push-ups or squats can be a foundation that leads to much more. Instead, you're told to go on extreme diets or do exercises I never heard about before (I think you can trust me that I've heard of a lot of exercises).

Better health isn't built on a foundation of complexity. It's about doing what you can every day, and then doing a little more the next day. That's called progressive resistance. Today you do one push-up, tomorrow you do two. It seems like such minor progress, but after a year when you zoom out, you see those tiny wins built into a giant vision.

Today, your brain is filled with overcomplicated details that make you stress about every meal, every rep, and many unnecessary supplements. It's time to shift away from that approach to something much more effective.

Before I became the greatest bodybuilder or an action star, I focused on building habits and routines. There's no way I could deadlift 700 pounds or become Mr. Olympia if I had to stress about everything I ate or followed plans that made me feel bad about myself. I created an unstoppable mindset that allowed me to unlock the unlimited potential of the human body. I believe this book can help do the same for you.

Today, everyone forgets that the first step to an unbreakable foundation is simple. And that's why I know this book can help so many people. It's a throwback to timeless principles with updated, science-backed recommendations to help you survive and thrive in today's environment. It isn't complicated. And it isn't negative.

I've known Adam for more than ten years. In addition to being one of the smartest people in nutrition I've met, he's the perfect person to blaze a better path that provides a more direct, realistic, and effective way to improve your health and mindset and achieve your goals.

We have every reason to be healthier than ever if we stop with the one-size-fits-all recommendations. Many of my favorite bodybuilders of all time followed very different plans than me. That is because lots of things work for different types of people. The key is finding the right tools that work for everyone and providing room for personalization.

I wanted to eat *kaiserschmarrn* and cherry pie and be the world's greatest bodybuilder. Your goals might differ, but the desire for healthy balance lives within us all. Consider this your guide to turning that dream into a reality.

If you embrace the lessons of *You Can't Screw This Up*, you'll build a more positive mindset and develop healthier habits. And that is the most powerful combination in the world.

—*Arnold Schwarzenegger*

INTRODUCTION

Hope

YOU ARE NOT ALONE.

That's the first thing you need to know before you dig into this book. Because if there's one thing I know, it's that millions of people feel just as stuck as you. At this point, dieting and—in fact—the whole wellness industry probably feels like a fraud. I'm not saying eating chicken and broccoli and working out six times per week won't get results. It's that the idea you're sold of "health" has painted a distorted reality that is breaking your mind and damaging your body.

We categorize health as a choice. And while you have a say in what you eat and how you exercise, the environment you live in and the endless options you're given make it hard to see the real problems. There are dozens of diets, each offering differing opinions, which means you never really feel confident that you're doing the right thing for your body. The one thing that appears clear is that you need to cut out everything that sounds delicious and follow meticulous plans that don't consider the best way to help you succeed. It's all about "one-size-fits-all" instead of considering your particular needs, preferences, and strengths. And when you don't follow these plans, you're shamed and blamed and told you don't care about your health.

At the same time, you're told that you shouldn't follow a plan that distorts your body image, creates stress about food, or makes you do things that aren't sustainable. And yet, most diets are anxiety-producing, frustration-generating, and feel like they were designed to expire after only a few weeks.

Add it all up, and the trillion-dollar wellness industry is built on a foundation of shortsightedness and conflict. The focus is on the body and rarely on the mind. But by ignoring your mind, you're missing the most important piece of lifestyle change, and—in doing so—you're creating the perfect recipe for failure and frustration. Because what you're told it takes to be healthy oftentimes adds more stress to your life and makes you feel worse. That combination makes it more likely that your new behaviors won't last, your results will stall or disappear, and you'll become more convinced that you're broken and need to go to extremes for a solution.

Sadly, for many in the wellness industry, it feels like that's the point. The worse you feel, the more desperate you become in your search for an answer, and the more willing you are to try something that, in your heart, doesn't feel right. You're being sold solutions that keep you buying answers rather than being given tools that solve problems and put you in control of your health.

This isn't a question about doing things that are good for your body or taking on new challenges. Prioritizing your health is the foundation of less disease, more vitality, and a higher quality of life. And, if you're reading this book and looking for a way to become healthier, then you realize something needs to change.

But, if you ask the average person what it takes to be fit, most will tell you it requires taste preferences you don't possess, foods that cost more money than you have, time you can't seem to find, and habits you haven't yet built. It's not that people don't want to be healthy, feel good, and have energy. It's that most people doubt that they can find a program that actually works for them in the long run.

That's probably why you're here—and why you're likely skeptical. You want to believe that this time will be different. But you're worried it's the same experience packaged differently. Just another plan that promises the world and only delivers if you're willing to sacrifice everything and suffer from mental and physical burnout. Because at some point, the more you repeat the "try, fail, try again" pattern of dieting, the more you're inclined to believe you are broken.

I'm here to give you hope that there is a different way.

I want you to see that the root of so many of your struggles is not what you've been told. For years, the conversation has focused on complex topics such as your broken metabolism, imbalanced hormones, and toxic foods. But what if I told you there's something bigger happening that's the real cause of all your health struggles? And no, I'm not talking about removing another food (no carb-phobia in this book), trying another detox, or only eating at certain times of day.

For decades, dieting has used unnecessary tactics to try and change you physically, and, in the process, those diets have broken you mentally. This approach has ruined how you look at food, painted an inaccurate picture of what it takes to be healthy, and created a vicious cycle of guilt, anxiety, and stress. The more it changes your mental outlook, the more you fall apart and suffer physically. Mix it all together and you've been served a shame cocktail that has overcomplicated nutrition and made you feel like you're always doing something wrong *and* never doing enough.

I'd argue that your experience with past diets is a big reason you're convinced it's unrealistic to find something that will work for your body because you've been programmed to restrict foods and punish yourself when you eat those "forbidden" options. And whether you realize it or not, all that restriction is just making you crave foods more, lessen your control over what you want to eat, and create more guilt and shame that can lead to overeating.

The feelings and frustrations that got you to this point are the same ones I've been helping people tackle for twenty years. At the heart of the issue are how these diets make you think and feel. It sounds something like:

I'm going to screw this up.

I've heard it again and again. In fact, when I led a group of five hundred people through this exact plan, so many people said the same thing I changed the book's title from *The Takeout Diet* (because I want people to know that eating takeout isn't a sin and can be a part of a healthy plan) to the title you see on the cover. It's a mantra that I believe will change your health for the better.

Repeat after me: You can't screw this up.

It's time to step away from plans that make you believe that perfectly normal behaviors—like eating takeout, having dessert, or missing workouts—are mistakes or the core of an unhealthy lifestyle. You can't mistreat your body, but shifting how you react to these behaviors is how you achieve amazing results. Most important, changing how you perceive yourself is the real secret to building better habits, feeling more in control, and finally upgrading your health.

The entire structure and strategy of diets are an illusion that would be easy to spot in any other scenario. Imagine if you were told you had one month to successfully complete a big project when, in reality, the project required four to six months to be done correctly. Also, you couldn't take off any days during the process and you needed to develop a new style of doing work that you'd never tried before. Naturally, you would burn out quickly, get sick, and fail at the task. And, if you repeated this process multiple times per year for many years on end, you'd probably end up believing something was wrong with *you*. Welcome to wellness: an impossible task that breaks you mentally and then physically.

It might not make sense yet, but what you desire starts with accepting that your health and the ability to change your body is not a personal failing. If you can do that, then you can walk away from the typical manipulative approach of the plans you've tried before and walk toward a new way of living that will deliver a much better outcome.

Right now, you're probably exhausted and hoping there's a different way to be healthy. I know the promises sound a little gimmicky, but this book isn't about tricks, hacks, or illusions. It's an antidote to all of the above. There is a global health crisis because we can't figure out how to make our bodies work for us. It's a paradox that defies all logic.

Healthcare is seemingly the only industry where endless resources and investments all result in worse outcomes. In the United States, the CDC estimates that more than $300 billion is spent cumulatively on diabetes, and yet the rate of diabetes has never been higher. You don't have to look far to realize there is an overwhelming number of people trying diets, while obesity rates continue to climb, eating disorders become more commonplace, and the supplement industry grows to billions of dollars without making a real difference.

I've worked with thousands of people who have built healthier habits, lost weight (and kept it off), and reclaimed control of their life and comfort with their bodies. My approach doesn't involve completely eliminating one specific food, micromanaging macronutrients, or worrying about toxins in foods. In fact, I'm going to suggest that you spend a little less time trying to figure out nutrition science and a little more time focused on behavioral change. Because if you want to stop the madness, it's time to recognize that you've been given the wrong tools for the job.

BREAK THE GLASS

Years ago, a windowpane almost ended my marriage.

Okay, that might be a slight exaggeration. But, at the time, it felt like everything might fall apart because of a seemingly impossible chore that created a little too much tension. If you're married or in a relationship, you know that some of the worst arguments are caused by an overblown, unresolved conflict.

When my wife and I moved into our current home, it wasn't your traditional buying experience. I never saw the property until after my wife purchased the house. I was busy traveling for work (much more on this soon), I trusted her, and before I was back from work, the house was under contract.

It was a beautiful home with lots of potential, but the previous owners hadn't taken good care of the place. The home needed a lot of love, renovation, and imagination to make it what we wanted it to be. And one room—a third-story loft—caused more trouble than the rest. It had everything you could want: vaulted ceilings, skylights, a bathroom, two closets, and enough space to put a huge office or a suite for our two young boys. There was just one problem: It also came with an eyesore.

The glass of the only window in the room was covered in kid's paint. This wasn't just any paint—it felt like it was immovable—and it was placed by the previous owner's daughter. The entire window was covered with her name written in every font possible: swiggles and circles, and black, yellow, blue, purple, and white (seriously, why so many colors?).

By the time that family had moved out, the daughter was in college, which means the paint had set for at least ten years. Like a bad tattoo after a drunken night out, the window drove my wife crazy. Home decor is her love language, and the window was unacceptable. The third floor was *her space*. She called it her "NBA" or "No Boys Allowed." It was her office, her creative space, and a place to enjoy a cocktail, read a book, or just have a little silence in a house of three boys. But, when you entered the room, the first thing you saw was that ugly window. And to complicate things, I'm not what you would call handy. Changing a lightbulb can be an adventure (hey, these hands were made for typing and deadlifts), but I desperately wanted to make her happy and clean the window.

I googled every solvent in the world. From Goo Gone to vinegar, rubbing alcohol to acetone (word to the wise: be careful with acetone!). I tried seemingly everything and nothing stood a chance against the paint. At one point, I joked I would just break the window and buy a new one. I didn't, but it might've been the best move, because the paint wasn't going anywhere, which means it was a pilot light for an argument at any moment. All you needed to do was flip the switch.

Fast-forward three years, and one day my wife and I were having a disagreement. And, as in all good marital battles, unresolved issues turned a small disagreement into a bonfire. The immortal paint on the window came up, and let's just say things got irrationally heated. (Let's be honest: I should've found a way to fix the issue, so her frustration was understandable.)

In a moment of desperation and frustration, I grabbed a razor blade I was using for crafts with the kids and headed upstairs. For a second—okay, maybe about five minutes—I thought about breaking the window. It was the only way.

Or was it?

Don't ask me how or why, but in that moment, I looked at the paint, then at the blade, then back at the paint, and I had an idea. "What if . . . this is so dumb . . . but, what if I used a knife on the glass?"

To you this might seem obvious, but to the guy who outsources all home fixes, this idea seemed dumb at best and dangerous at worst. And yet, this was not the time to overthink anything. I raised the blade into the air, and instead of trying to smash the glass, I started chipping away like a madman. I was convinced I would scratch the window, crack the glass, or—most likely—lose a finger.

Instead of the expected disaster, I was delighted. Piece by piece, the paint started coming off. The more I understood how to use the blade, the easier the job became. I saw better angles, found weaknesses in the paint that once seemed impenetrable, and embraced a strategy that made it seem as if the impossible mess would soon be gone.

After three years alternating fruitless effort and (ultimately not) benign neglect, I undid all the damage in two hours, and the window was as good as new. I remember when my wife came upstairs, still reeling from the argument, and the mood changed completely when she saw the spotless window.

You might see where I'm going with this.

The paint is your complicated relationship with your health.
The solvents are the traditional approaches to dieting and exercise.
And the blade is this book.

Many of you have probably been struggling to figure out your health for much longer than three years. Maybe you've never found anything that worked. Or, like so many, you've tried a diet or workout, lost some weight, and gained it all back. And you might think you've turned over every stone, but you've likely just been using another variation of the same old paint remover. Even if you had success—many people *do* lose weight—the pounds always seem to come back. You don't want a temporary fix, you want something that works for good and makes you feel like you actually hit reset and resolved whatever was making it hard for you to be healthier.

If you're being honest with yourself, it's time to find a new tool to undo the damage of your dieting past and try something that leaves you feeling confident that you truly fixed the issue. The fix isn't another superfood or elimination diet. I want you to step back for a second and think about those "different" plans. You've been programmed to believe any (or all) of the following:

- Your body is stuck and needs to be reset. It could be your metabolism, hormones, or your gut.
- Scientists have discovered the one type of food you need to remove and—if it's removed—suddenly everything will be better.

- Scientists have discovered the one type of food—or perfect breakdown of nutrients—you need to eat, and if you follow the plan to a T, everything will be fine.

And if you're not a fan of diets, you might just believe that genetics determine everything, so why bother?

No matter which option you select, the road to better health feels like it's designed to work for the minority of people who are willing to adhere to a strict set of rules, and the rest are left to figure it out or suffer. That's not an opinion. Throughout this book, you'll see research that suggests people who go on diets tend to have worse outcomes than those who don't. It's not that diets can't work, it's that many of the most popular approaches don't address foundational issues. If you're focused on eliminating inflammation from your diet, but you don't know how to feel satisfied with a meal unless it's something "unhealthy," I can promise you that the results won't be what you want. It's like using a roll of paper towel to fix a broken pipe. You might clean up the mess, but eventually, the puddle of water is coming right back and could lead to a flood. You haven't been taught how to avoid falling back into the old habits, especially when you're stressed and busy. If that feels like your life, it becomes easier to understand why the journey to feeling and looking the way you want is paved in pain, shame, guilt, and unsatisfying results.

The wellness industry ends up making you feel bad about how you eat and the way you live. Whether it's intentional or not, the outcome is psychological warfare that breaks you down instead of builds you up. And that difference matters much more than whether you eat more or less carbs. While there's been some progress about acceptance of health at different sizes, if you want to make changes, the plans are still built around one extreme or another, and the all-or-none belief is a dangerous psychological mentality. Once that mindset takes hold, it finds its way into your daily behaviors and makes it incredibly hard to eat well and move frequently.

We know from obesity research that failure to lose weight can lead to significant distress that affects self-perception and well-being.[1] Once that happens, it makes it harder to shift behaviors that can improve your health.

And those mental shifts are not limited to people suffering from obesity; we are all vulnerable.

The biggest adjustment you need is one that takes you away from strict rules and trades them for more effective tools.

It's about having practical plans that are desired for the chaotic nature of real life and abandoning plans that are fundamentally created around concepts of perfection, restriction, or punishment. And, most importantly, it's about building a pattern of success so you can progress to different levels of healthy living without thinking it's an all-or-nothing relationship. Add it all up, and you won't just end up with fitness and nutrition suggestions that fit your lifestyle, you'll also change the way you see yourself and improve your ability conquer conflict. And that's the adjustment that matters most.

This book is different than anything I've seen out there. Sure, I'll share studies that explain better ways to eat. But you won't waste your time debating whether you need to cut carbs or fat. Because, as you're about find out, you can eat both.

There will be meal plans and food lists, but they won't look like the food lists you've seen before. Foods like bread, potatoes, and rice won't be forbidden. And you won't have to stress about the amount of time between meals or if you can eat breakfast or have a meal at night. You'll be able to eat takeout and have dessert. (It won't be only as a reward, and you won't need to compensate with punishment.)

You'll have workouts and exercises. But they will be shorter than you're used to, and the movements won't be complicated.

You'll learn from doctors, scientists, and researchers. But, more importantly, you'll learn life-changing lessons from those who have mastered self-improvement. I spent the early part of my career, before I dedicated my life to helping people improve their health, focused on behavioral change. I have a degree in psychology, worked as a researcher in social psychology labs at the University of Colorado, and learned that the biggest barriers to physiological change tend to start with the mind. It's cliché to say "where the mind goes the body follows," but it's also true . . . which is why diets that break you mentally on the path to improving you physically are fatally flawed.

Throughout the years, I saw that the best trainers and nutritionists would struggle in their quest to support long-term change for their clients. Part of this is because day-to-day life and the food environment doesn't make it easy. The other part is that their approach was missing the most important piece: Recommending the best foods and exercises without considering someone's mindset or habits is like providing high-quality fuel for a car with no engine.

I've studied the work of those who have built the strongest engines that support healthier lifestyles. People like habits expert James Clear, vulnerability queen Brené Brown, and Ryan Holiday, the man who popularized the ancient philosophy of stoicism for modern times. These individuals and so many others have unlocked what it takes to change your current state into something much better. It's ridiculous that their advice hasn't been applied to the most complicated change of all—improving health. And that's where I come in. I applied their proven methods of change to nutrition, fitness, and overall wellness, so you can finally stop living in neutral and reach your goals.

The approach in this book sees eating and exercise as behavioral adjustments—not about needing higher education in nutrition and exercise physiology.

You'll still learn about better foods to eat and effective exercises. In fact, I'll outline the foods I'm convinced are doing the most damage, the ones that will keep you more satisfied, and a method of exercising that delivers consistent results. Those details will be the background noise, because you can eat much more than you've been told, and there are many ways to build an effective workout program. You just need a stress-free, confidence-inspiring plan to pull it all together.

Instead of the doom and gloom statistics like, "Only five percent of people maintain weight loss," you'll find countless stories of people who have transformed their lives for good. And they didn't do it by breaking the bank or sacrificing their lifestyle.

When I talked to people like you—including those five hundred people who tested the program in this book—it reaffirmed that the last thing you need is the only thing you've been given. So, say goodbye to super restrictive diet plans, endless rules, and complicated meals. It's time to abandon the plans that don't feel realistic, even if you've been told they are what you "must" do.

That doesn't mean you'll be spending your days eating comfort foods and magically transforming. If that's your expectation, go get a refund (sorry, publisher!). That's not what this book is about. Change brings discomfort. This is a good thing. You were built to adapt and turn tribulation into transformation. The magic is in how you go from your current state to the one you desire without falling into the same patterns of the past. (Spoiler alert: It doesn't consist of restricting everything and living in a constant state of stress.)

HOW TO USE THIS BOOK

You've probably read books that felt like they could've been a ten-page guide. That's the last thing I wanted to create. I want to give you helpful recommendations, but also recognize that each and every one of you has different needs and experiences. I structured this book to meet you where you are. There are four main sections.

PART 1 IS REQUIRED READING. *Sure, you can skip to the eating plans, but you're going to miss out on everything that will make them work for you. Every great structure needs a rock-solid foundation, and that's Part 1. If you're going to get any value out of this book, then you must understand how you can start playing a different game and see infinitely better results, and that starts with rethinking everything about nutrition, fitness, and overall wellness—and putting a new emphasis on your self-perception and how you react to perceived failures.*

PART 2 IS ABOUT ASSESSMENT AND CONTROL. *You'll learn all the different ways that diets fail, and how to not fall for the same old tricks. It might seem like a Paleo Diet is completely different from an intermittent fasting protocol, but they use a surprisingly similar method.*
That's not to say either plan is bad (they're not); but the reason so many of these plans don't work is that they don't address how you end up back in the same frustrating position. The name of the game is ending frustration and stress and adding flexibility, control, and results. Depending on where you're most out of

control, you can dive into those aspects of Part 2 to find out whether you need more help understanding the role of stress, or genetics, or your environment.

PART 3 IS ABOUT FREEDOM. *It's practical advice that you can apply to your everyday life. You'll learn why most diet rules are overrated and why you just need a few boundaries that help you find foods that work with your preference and work well for your body. And yes, that includes eating takeout without feeling like you're going off the plan and doing damage.*

PART 4 INCLUDES WORKOUTS AND EXERCISE ROUTINES. *These plans will support everything you learn in this book. If you already have a workout you love, it can work perfectly fine with the nutrition guidelines. These routines are more about efficiency and flexibility, so you don't have to live in the gym. I designed the program to offer a minimum effective dose—workouts that are all 15 to 30 minutes—to help you get the most results from the least amount of time.*

A REASON TO BELIEVE

If you've spent your life thinking you need to eat bland meals, can't touch sugar, and avoid restaurants, then you've come to the right place. If you want more freedom and more positive changes, this book is for you.

Some people will think I'm offering a gimmicky way to eat bad food, but that's only because the nutrition industry keeps selling you one lie after another. This is a step away from the only game you know. I don't care if you choose to eat takeout or avoid dessert, or whether you prefer an omnivorous or vegan diet. As you'll see, those decisions don't determine whether you can succeed. What really matters is resetting your mind, reprogramming what you think is healthy, learning how to co-exist (not fight against) the food environment, and avoiding the guilt that sends you spiraling.

This book is a guide that will help you make healthy living work for your busy life, while helping you navigate food temptation without anxiety and stress. If this book does anything, I hope it helps you drown out the noise so you know exactly what will work for you. Because extreme measures are not necessary for great health outcomes. Instead of fear, this book emphasizes . . .

- PROVIDING A PLAN THAT'S DESIGNED FOR REAL LIFE. Whether you eat takeout or enjoy a glass of wine, these should *not* feel like guilty pleasures or just be reserved for "cheat day."
- HAVING AN EXERCISE PLAN THAT FITS INTO YOUR SCHEDULE AND DELIVERS RESULTS, even if you have only twenty minutes and need to exercise at home.
- UNDERSTANDING ONCE AND FOR ALL WHY YOU STILL STRUGGLE TO LOSE WEIGHT. It's a combination of the restrictive plan and your *reaction* to missteps that aren't really mistakes.
- CREATING A NEW FRAMEWORK THAT MAKES IT EASIER TO NAVIGATE THE REASONS WEIGHT GAIN FEELS INEVITABLE (so that it is no longer an inevitability). This starts with understanding you don't need to avoid every type of food you enjoy.
- FEELING SEEN. Struggling with your health is frustrating. It doesn't matter if you want to lose 10 or 100 pounds, or if you just want to move and feel better. As my wife says, "There's no hierarchy of pain." I want to meet you where you are, so you can have the tools you need to live the life you want.
- GIVING YOU HOPE. After all this time, I know that most people think they can't change no matter what they do. It becomes a self-fulfilling prophecy. Let's fix that. You are not destined to be unhealthy. Because—as I'll help you understand—you need to believe that you are healthy. The problem isn't who you are, it's how you've been told to live.

This book is personal. It's a bit controversial because it focuses on the mental, emotional, and behavioral impact most diet books prefer to ignore. It's an explanation of stress, real life, broken promises, and new realities. If the old way was about restriction, this new way is about abundance, transparency, and a plan that will keep working in spite of the fact that you'll never be perfect or completely compliant.

It's probably not what you expect, and it's also the most effective way to permanently leave the vicious cycle of dieting. Instead of starts and stops, you'll build an unbreakable foundation that will help you dramatically transform your health, rebuild your relationship with food, and enjoy your meals more than ever before.

I don't profess to have all the answers, but I did have a mission while writing this book: Put an end to the short-term plans that require extreme discomfort and sacrifice and *don't deliver long-term results*. What you're about to learn requires open-mindedness because it challenges much of what you've been told. And, if I'm being honest, that's my favorite part of the book. You need something dramatically different to give you the good health you deserve.

I wrote *You Can't Screw This Up* because I don't want you to settle for another restrictive, miserable eating plan. I wanted you to have a blueprint that would help you thrive in any situation, season, or scenario. You should be able to live the life you want without living a life you can't stand. When that happens, you'll see those past obstacles are opportunities. And when you use the right tools, what once felt permanently broken—your health, confidence, and sanity—will finally be fixed for the better.

YOU CAN'T SCREW THIS UP

PART 1

THE UNBREAKABLE FOUNDATION

Chapter 1

SO EASY IT'S HARD TO FAIL

What would it look like if this was easy?

I'M NOT EXAGGERATING WHEN I say this question has helped me solve complex problems better than anything else I've tried in my life. And I hope that you find it has the same seemingly mythical powers for curing whatever has caused you so much frustration with your nutrition, fitness, and overall wellness.

For about five years, I was the de facto chief marketing officer for Tim Ferriss. You might know Tim from his bestselling books like *The 4-Hour Body*, *The 4-Hour Workweek*, or *Tools of Titans*, or maybe you've listened to his insanely popular podcast, *The Tim Ferriss Show*. Millions love him and many others hate him because he's not afraid to share polarizing or controversial ideas and opinions. No matter what you might know, to me, he's the guy who changed my perspective on wellness without ever spending much time talking to me about diets or workouts. It's not how Tim ate or exercised that made me better at helping others; in fact, we disagree on many things about nutrition. It's how he approached complex problems.

Tim's brilliant. I learned more during my time working with him than at any other point in my life, whether in school, graduate education, or the working world. And the most powerful takeaway he gave me was that he asks questions that force you to think differently about a situation. Much like realizing I needed a blade to solve the window issue, Tim understands—

maybe better than anyone—that when you feel stuck, the best thing you can do is not grind through but stop and consider, *"What would it look like if this was easy?"*

We are trained to think that everything must be a struggle. The health industry thrives on making it seem that "if it tastes good or feels good, then it must be bad for you." (By that definition, clearly no one thinks sex is healthy, but I digress.) We wear pain like a badge of honor. We celebrate not eating or training so hard that you puke, and we cast judgment on anyone who enjoys sugar (even though everyone enjoys it, whether or not they choose to eat it). We share pictures on social media of doing cold plunges or getting IV therapy, but we don't think to celebrate an outdoor walk or a call to a friend. That's because the perception of what it takes to be healthy is very far from the scientifically proven foundations you need.

As we'll discuss, discomfort is often a part of self-improvement. But discomfort and complexity are not the same things. And there's nothing that says you should be uncomfortable all the time. As you'll learn, *expanding your comfort zone—not abandoning it—is the secret* to creating new behaviors that last. And that means you can find easier routes on complex journeys. It just requires looking at the map differently.

That brings me back to Tim and his special talent. When I worked for him, whenever something seemed too complicated, he would ask me the "what would it look like . . ." question. Coming up with the answer was always incredibly hard, but only because I was forced to consider things that were counterintuitive, unconventional, or experimental.

The idea of "making hard easy" aligns beautifully with the psychology of behavioral change. This field is dedicated to helping people master difficult, complex behaviors, whether abandoning addiction or losing weight. And, for the most part, the research suggests that if you want to develop a new behavior—such as eating healthier—the best way is to *make it so easy that it's hard to fail.* [1]

Read that line again because it's different than what you've been told. In traditional goal setting, you focus on ambitious goals and outcomes. But, in behavioral change, you want the process and tasks themselves to be easy. Fewer tasks. Less complication. More action.

Once the tasks become routine, you add new tasks and they also feel easy. The magic here is that the second, third, and fourth tiers of tasks *feel* easy. However, in reality, if you were to start at the second, third, or fourth level, it would feel impossible. *Because easy is relative to your current state.* Multiplying five by seven is a brain bender for a four year old but child's play for a fourteen year old.

And that's the beauty of making it hard to fail. If you keep starting with the concept of easy, getting good at something, and then progressing, you can take on hard challenges and accomplish amazing outcomes. The key is always keeping it easy relative to where you are, not where you want to be.

Making the hard feel easy so you can embrace discomfort and become better is the North Star of this book. Over the years of helping people, I always came back to that question, until it clicked, and an obstacle became an opportunity.

THE OBSTACLE IS THE WAY

The Obstacle Is the Way is a book by Ryan Holiday about stoicism. You might wonder what a bunch of ancient philosophers can teach you about dieting. The answer is a lot of guidance you badly need. I'd argue that a stoic approach to dieting is the solution to our broken diet culture.

Stoicism boosts happiness by providing an effective way of handling the hurdles in your life. A core stoic principle is that you don't control the world around you—you control how you respond to it. If you apply this to nutrition, instead of pretending that you can remove the obstacles that make it hard to eat healthily–such as takeout food and dessert–it's better to embrace them as part of life. Food is everywhere. Unless you decide to isolate yourself completely, you're going to be seeing many different delicious food options. That's why it's important to learn how to be comfortable in your environment.

It's been great that no foods are off limits. That is a huge psychological ease to me and the family. In the past I've tried every diet under the sun—South Beach, Paleo, keto, IF, Renegade—and while they all "work" for a while, it's

easy to fall off and then get discouraged about starting again. With yours, there is no falling off, so that eliminates the guilt and self-defeatism that comes with most diets. I've lost weight, gained muscle, and can see myself doing this for a very long time!
—Michael A.

In *The Obstacle Is the Way,* Holiday says,

Overcoming obstacles is a discipline of three critical steps. It begins with how we look at our specific problems, our attitude or approach; then the energy and creativity with which we actively break them down and turn them into opportunities; finally, the cultivation and maintenance of an inner will that allows us to handle defeat and difficulty.

It's three interdependent, interconnected, and fluidly contingent disciplines: Perception, Action, and the Will.

The stoics didn't have to worry about a minefield of diet obstacles and brain-altering food. Some of these problems you know about and others might be a total surprise. We'll cover how to work around every hurdle, but the most important lesson is realizing you can't—and don't need to—avoid every single one . . . a task that would be virtually impossible in today's food environment anyway.

Each time you eat something that's forbidden, the first domino drops, with everything else not far behind. That's why a touch of logical stoic philosophy is exactly what's needed to make sense of our illogical diet plans. Why fight the system when you can learn to coexist?

THE MAGIC PILL

Have you ever been told that one change will miraculously make everything better? If so, you've experienced the magic pill approach to health. It looks like an answer to the "What would it look like if this was easy?" question, but it's really a wolf in sheep's clothing because most often the change in question is removing things like carbs, sugar, or eating at night—which aren't easy at all for most people. The magic pill proposition allows you to win a battle against one food only to lose the war on better health.

You can spot the flaw by looking at the patterns of diets over the last forty years. Popular diet suggestions tend to look something like these . . .

Fat makes you fat.
Carbs make you fat.
Eating breakfast makes you fat.
Eating too much too late at night makes you fat.
Gluten makes you fat.
Dairy makes you fat.
Non-Paleo foods make you fat.
Inflammation makes you fat.
Disrupted hormones make you fat.
High blood sugar makes you fat.
High-glycemic carbs make you fat.

The list goes on, but you get the idea. Diets love to focus on what could cause weight gain. That's like giving a list of all the ways you can run out of money. Just because you can spend it, doesn't mean you're going broke. How you grow your wealth depends on how you save and invest, regardless of how much you make. Do you have a savings account? Investments? Are you living within your means?

Food is the same way. There are many things that can cause you to gain weight, and all of them are connected to eating too many calories. Your job is to determine a plan that makes it easier for you to make good decisions that keep you from feeling nutritionally bankrupt.

It's easy to see when you make or lose money. But unlike finance, it's harder to know what causes weight gain. And, while you have a scale, it's harder to measure diets that are working because you might be doing everything right but the scale might not be moving. Or, it goes down and then back up, and you think something is wrong. That's why it's important to see the bigger picture and not overreact to small, normal fluctuations. It's more about staying the course rather than constantly taking detours.

No one food in one dose will cause health problems (or cure them). If you want to become healthier, you must stop stressing every single food you eat. Yes, you need to limit the amount of overprocessed foods you eat. And you'll learn how. Beyond that, it's about simplifying the way you approach food.

You've been taught to worry about fixing your metabolism and your hormones. Or to avoid different types of foods that might cause inflammation. These are all a sleight of hand. When you look at the research, you see that sugar isn't fattening on its own (every gram of sugar is only 4 calories). Carbs won't make you fat as long as you're not overeating total calories. An inflammatory response is completely normal—and healthy—as long as the inflammation doesn't stay elevated. Blood sugar spikes are also normal and have no impact on hunger or hormones as long as they don't stay elevated. So why are you paying money to wear a continuous glucose monitor and react to every fluctuation?

Most health barriers aren't removed with perfection or optimization. They need the right combination of effective and practical. Living a healthier life is about aligning friction with relief. Paving a path you're not ready to walk only creates a less bumpy road; it doesn't mean you'll get to your target destination.

You might be thinking, "Okay, but what does that mean in real life? What should I change?" And the answer is to stop trying to hack your health. Your body is made up of wildly complex mechanisms that can't be solved by removing a food group. It's less about, "Is there one single food I should eliminate?" and more, "What can I eat to feel full *and* not have intense cravings and feel stressed?"

That's how you make this easy. You stop trying to play armchair nutrition scientist, and lean into the habits and behaviors you can understand and apply. That means eating foods that fill you up so you don't have cravings, and enjoying some of your favorite foods so you don't feel completely restricted. When you do that, the biology of your body—both physiologically and psychologically—takes care of itself. We'll discuss more about how you can pull off this one-two punch successfully. But, know this: More hunger satisfaction and less food restriction are the first step to easy success.

CONTROL THE CONTROLLABLE

A popular saying in stoicism is *amor fati* or "love of fate." Translated loosely, it's the idea that we do not have control over our outcomes; instead, we can only control our actions and how we react in any given situation.

The conversation about weight loss and gain usually focuses on what you need to eat. But, often, the biggest problem isn't knowing what foods are healthy.

Tamar Haspel is an award-winning journalist who has covered nutrition for decades. And if you ask her why it's so hard to lose weight, the answer is clear to her.

"When I talk to people who are struggling with their weight and I ask, 'What does a good food day look?' they can easily identify good and bad foods. The problem isn't education, it's temptation. We encounter temptation everywhere we turn. The reason the medicalization of obesity has failed is that most of the time we overeat because we are tempted. It's not always because we are hungry. And when we eat, we feel guilty and eat more. When 75 percent of the system can't navigate the system, you have to look hard at the system itself."

The key is being aware of the temptation and making it easier for you to eat without perpetual guilt. Life is complicated and messy and rarely goes the way you want or expect. In a perfect world, you would cook every meal (and have plenty of time to do so), would never have cravings for foods that are loaded with calories, and get great sleep every night (while not stressing about why you can't fall asleep). But that's not how it works. You need more flexibility so you can adjust to real life. That means having a plan that supports you during the days when you don't have time to cook because work is breathing down your neck, you want sugar because your in-laws are driving you crazy, and you can't sleep because you're burned out, your kids are crying, and your carb-starved diet has you going to bed hungry every night.

On the hardest days, it's highly unlikely you're going to take an hour to prepare a meal when a few swipes on your phone will give you what you need. And, when that happens, you shouldn't feel like you failed. But most meal plans don't account for days when mac and cheese is the only option.

That's why you need a plan that provides flexible boundaries for the stressed-out, chaotic days when you eat a less-healthy option. And, more importantly, when you can't be "perfect," there's no reason to think you've ruined the entire week, which means you don't respond to those moments by going off the rails and eating everything.

You can't screw this up if it's hard to screw up. And when it comes to dieting, it's important to realize that most "screw ups" are not mistakes at all. They are expected variations you can sustain because your plan—and your body—is built to withstand them. Much like a good glass window can handle a carefully handled blade scraping off paint, your body can handle occasional meals where every food isn't the definition of health.

If you can "turn on the lights" and see that you don't need to control every meal and all the chaos of your day, then you can find your way. This means avoiding plans that are built for controlled environments that look nothing like your real life. Plans that disregard the very elements that make you a human are designed to fail.

This is where it's good to focus on what you control, while embracing when you have a little less control. I'm going to recommend you cook more often and eat more nutritious foods. But, you don't need to be perfect with either of those goals. And, if you understand that you *won't* always eat in a way that would make a dietitian applaud, then you're starting to understand this approach.

Part of seeing the obstacle clearly is realizing you need a plan built for chaos and unpredictability. You need something that feels like it understands your life. Remember how I started the book by saying you can't screw this up? A diet that treats normal life (such as ordering takeout) as a mistake is a diet you want to avoid.

Most people understand how to differentiate healthy from unhealthy foods. Research shows that almost everyone knows fruits and vegetables are good, and fast food is not so good. You don't need another grocery list of foods you hate or to feel shamed for your love of dessert. Sure, a plan like that can be effective . . . but only if you follow it consistently.

You need tools that make life easier and also help you make good choices when stressed and stretched for time. Most important, you need a plan that makes it easier to eat foods you enjoy *and will* fill you up so you don't keep eating and eating without feeling satisfied.

That means understanding which foods are most addicting, why habits are hard to change, and how to turn your weaknesses into strengths. All three of these skills will make your life much easier—with a lot less stress—than trying to figure out if low-carb is better than vegan.

DIETS THAT FOCUS ON REMOVAL, RESTRICTION, AND INFLEXIBLE RULES HAVE VERY LOW LONG-TERM SUCCESS RATES. Good plans are built around timeless principles that allow you to adapt and adjust so it's hard to fail. Great plans help you understand that mistakes can be tolerated, there is slack in the system, and punishment is not the way to get back on track. The focus isn't as much about removing things as it is about adding support so you don't break down mentally and physically as your body changes.

When you try to improve your nutrition, you typically build a shaky foundation. These are the faulty principles you want to *avoid*:

- EXTREME SACRIFICE IS THE ONLY WAY: The changes you think you need are not the changes that will lead to long-term success.
- MORE COMPLEXITY = MORE RESULTS: Most diets mandate adjustments that are so complex and cumbersome that they create stress, frustration, and anxiety. These plans are made of glass and not designed for the normal chaos of day-to-day life, which means perfectly "regular" adjustments are considered mistakes that send you off course. If it feels like you can easily fall off the wagon, you're on the wrong ride. It's the twenty-first century. Why is anyone using a wagon?
- DIETING IS A GAME OF CHECKERS: Checkers is basic. You move forward and backward. You gain weight and lose weight, and when you're not losing weight, it means you're doing something wrong. None of this is true. Diets don't prepare you for how your body changes when you *do* lose weight. Lots of people lose weight. Almost all of them gain it back. And it's no surprise because your body adjusts as you drop weight, so if you're not taking the right steps to lose the weight in the first place, the rebound can easily knock you down.

If you can accept that these three flaws exist, then you're already in position to succeed. The last ten years of research has made clear that your brain plays a key role in your ability to be healthy, lose weight, and have a better relationship with food. Diets go wrong because goals and expectations are misaligned. You only need extreme measures for extreme results. And by extreme results, I mean the top percentile of physical health.

If you need to lose 5 pounds to get yourself into a healthier body, you don't need extremes. If you need to lose 100 pounds to get yourself into a healthier body, you also don't need extremes. Because in both situations, you're trying to establish improved health, not something very few ever accomplish, such a single-digit body fat. While the path is longer for the person who needs to lose 100 pounds, the journey is similar, and the best path is paved with consistency. For your behaviors to be consistent, they can't start with extremes.

Oddly enough, most healthy people—the ones who have figured out how to maintain a healthy weight, exercise, and eat well—don't feel like their habits and behaviors are a burden. That's because they've progressed to the point where their actions aren't a strain. Every step you take toward health shouldn't feel impossible.

When I was in my late teens and early twenties, I was a ski instructor for Vail Resorts. The first few lessons were designed to create comfort. We would start with simple balancing drills that the students could master. After that, we'd progress to shifting their weight and making turns. Eventually, we'd go down runs, selecting steeper trails, and adding in bigger challenges like moguls. Some people wanted to become experts, and others were just happy being able to go down easier runs, have fun, and be confident.

Healthy eating is similar. Just like I would teach people to stand on their skis without falling over before going on runs, you need to master your balance with eating and your schedule. Only after you've checked off easier tasks should you need to decide if you want extremes, and—at that point—you'll be healthier and can determine how you want to continue to progress . . . or maybe you're happy where you are.

To do something for a long period of time, you need it—on some level—to be enjoyable. If you've read any diet book or article, you've likely heard many variations that explain why your struggles are "not your fault," and that the real reason you haven't succeeded yet is because of some new dietary problem. But it doesn't address the way you feel on these diets and what it does to the quality of your life.

Eventually, happiness matters. You care about being healthy, losing weight, and looking and feeling better. But, if you're miserable and unhappy while achieving this goal, you'll still feel like you've lost; and the behaviors you adopted to make those changes will be abandoned because you're looking out for your primary need—enjoying your life!

On the surface, this shouldn't be so hard. Venture capitalists are dumping money into billion-dollar companies that build diets based on your DNA and tell you what to eat based on fluctuations in your blood glucose. Everything is built around finding the exact foods you need to eat or remove. It's about timing your days around meals, avoiding takeout and desserts, and building a "lifestyle."

But do these diets ever ask what style of life you want? Do they consider the impact on your mental health? Do these diets even care about how you feel each time you're forced to overhaul everything without being met where you are?

You get one body. And, your health—including nutrition, fitness, and mental health—is the best investment you can make. And it's about time you got a better ROI for your time, money, and energy.

EMBRACE THE OBSTACLE

> Striving to be the best is a mistake. It creates an illusion of an endpoint—and a delusion that you can only succeed by beating others. Striving to be better shifts the focus from victory to mastery. You're competing with your past self and raising the bar for your future self.
> —Adam Grant

Instead of feeling like you must remove obstacles in your way, it's time to embrace them. The reason you struggle so much is that you don't have much control over the things that are most frustrating. Yes, you can remove certain foods from your diet, but until you understand that our food environment makes it harder to be healthy, it'll be difficult to build a plan that actually works. It's far more effective to adapt to your environment rather than create a new one.

Too many diets suggest that if you adjust the diet dial just right, then you'll unlock a faster metabolism, anti-aging benefits, and better health. Rarely do they discuss the collateral damage in your pursuit of dietary perfection. Good health does not require expensive biohacking or stress-inducing precision. If the endless assault of information makes you question everything you eat, that's when you know it's a problem.

You can optimize everything but if your quality of life is more stressful and you're unhappy, are you *really* healthier? This applies to a lot of things in life: When you find a good fit, you know it. You don't need to convince yourself otherwise.

> I've tried many diets and with most of them I gain the weight back. Stress plays a big part in my exercise and eating. Life gets busy and I stop doing what I need to do.
>
> I'm really enjoying the program. It's not stressful for me at all. Workouts take 30 minutes, and the simplified guidelines have made it very hard for me to overeat. My wife is eating better with me and has commented on how much more energy she has. I have four- and six-year-old daughters and they keep me going. I have had more energy and have been a lot happier since starting the program.
>
> —*Andrew B.*

It's time to reframe what it means to be healthy. "Perfection" should be measured by how well a diet plan makes it easy for you to eat better without losing your mind, not whether you can follow every last detail.

Your success isn't determined by the number of superfoods in your diet or whether you fast for fourteen or sixteen hours. What you need are tools designed to help you achieve outcomes. This includes things like feeling full after you eat, having energy, and getting the nutrition your body needs to function, while considering your budget, lifestyle, and food preferences. It's far more effective to focus on the outcomes and use methods that create less friction in your life. That's what real health looks like, and what creates a foundation that can withstand unpredictability.

One bad meal or an extra dessert will not cause you to spiral as long as you can see your actions for what they are and fall back on the habits and tools. The goal is to put yourself in the situations you've always avoided and learn how to not only survive but thrive. If you can believe you can eat well within the current food environment, then you don't need to diet again.

The only certainty about life is change and obstacles. You can try to build a fortress, or you can become a superball and learn to bounce off everything because you were built for it. If you can see obstacles differently, that's when food will create less stress. You'll have more control because you won't need to control everything. And you'll see opportunities to live your life and be healthy in scenarios you once thought you had to avoid.

CLOSE THE GAP

To prevent yourself from repeating the same mistakes that have led to disappointing outcomes, I want you to start at the end. That's when the problems with every diet become clear. When you combine this framework with stoicism, it's an unbeatable combination for building an effective plan that won't easily fall apart.

Remember when I talked about the beauty of Tim Ferriss's "What if" question? So much of this thought process is about forcing yourself to see things differently. The beginning of anything is the honeymoon stage. Hope is plentiful, motivation is limitless, and you're willing to believe that this time will be different.

But, in the end, it's an entirely different story. You're frustrated and anxious and usually doing everything possible to prevent yourself from quitting. By the end, you're dreading the inevitable. Whether you lost weight or not, made big changes or subtle shifts, in your heart you know that you can't maintain the pace and pressure. And that means the progress you made will disappear. The weight will come back. And, eventually, you'll have to try another diet, starve on another detox, or invest in another supplement. This ending sucks. But, if you know the bad way a diet can end, you can use this to your advantage.

The idea of working backward on a problem is called inversion. If you can invert your journey and start at your *undesired* state, then you can avoid the missteps that have led you down the same frustrating path every time you try to improve your health. This might seem like an awful way to start a new wellness plan. You want positive vibes and visions of success. But in reality, starting from a place you want to avoid will help you find the path you've been looking for.

Inversion isn't about preparing to fail. It's a better way to plan to succeed. When you invert the process, you can ask the questions that really matter.

Here's what I want you to do next. Below are six questions. Make sure you answer all of them—write them down in a journal or log them in a note on your phone. They will be your guide to a new outcome.

- What happened the last time a nutrition plan didn't work for me?
- How am I likely to fail as a healthier eater?
- What really upsets me when I start a new diet?
- When am I most likely to struggle with the plan?
- What are the types of foods I always desire that don't work for most diets?
- When do I get hungriest?

These questions allow honest conversations that will help you stop wasting time and start doing the things that are more likely to benefit you. More importantly, they'll help you see a better way to get the results you want if you're willing to learn from past experiences and learn what types of programs have led to less-than-ideal outcomes.

The gap between where you are and where you want to be is called frustration. The best way to eliminate frustration is a combination of education and action.

This is not the end of dieting. It's not a promise to solve all your problems. Instead, it's a validation of your frustration. An explanation of why things haven't worked. And a new approach that will remove many of the previous barriers and provide you with a few competitive advantages to upgrade your health for good.

CHAPTER SUMMARY

- Good health doesn't have to be complicated. Think about fewer tasks, more action, and confidence.
- Step away from "magic pill" thinking. Avoiding a single food (unless you have a food allergy or sensitivity) is not the answer. And yes, that includes sugar, too (there is a place for it).
- Accept that you will have stressful, difficult days when you won't eat perfectly, and that doesn't mean you can't be healthy. The best plan is built to include these types of days without stress and guilt.

Chapter 2

THE DIET GAME IS FIXED

What gets us into trouble is not what we don't know. It's what we know for sure that just ain't so.
—*Mark Twain*

IF YOU THINK DIETING is bad today, please step into my time machine. We will travel to the early twentieth century, when a different type of fat loss pill was all the rage. These earliest diet pills didn't even mess with your metabolism with a mix of caffeine and ephedra (because even back then they knew you couldn't create that big of a boost). Instead, the pills would plant a tapeworm egg in your body. When that egg hatched, a little baby tapeworm would dine on whatever you were feeding your body. Sure, the effectiveness of tapeworms eating your calories was completely hypothetical and wildly dangerous, but at least you could still eat . . . right?

Not to be outdone in the department of terrible ideas, the Prolinn Diet appeared in the 1970s and brought a new spin to daily starvation (what some people today might call intermittent fasting). The diet satisfied your tastebuds with a 400-calorie meal replacement consisting of slaughterhouse byproducts such as horns, hooves, and tendons (they lost me at byproducts).

If animal byproducts aren't your jam, maybe you would've preferred the Kimkins Diet. Like the tapeworm diet, Kimkins was all about giving you a way to lose weight without sweating calories–but without the whole issue of purposely growing a parasite. Instead, you could eat to your heart's content and offset those meals by loading up with enough laxatives to, well . . . you get the idea.

These diets may make keto look a little less threatening, but they all speak to the same issue. We are a little too obsessed with weight, and we tend to go to extremes to change the number on the scale. That's not to say weight gain isn't stressful or problematic. Most major diseases are directly related to how much body fat you carry. But obsessing about your weight is not the best way to change it. And working endlessly to burn the calories you eat doesn't work the way you've been led to believe.

THE "MOVE MORE, EAT LESS" LIE

When anthropologists try to understand the healthy behaviors of different cultures, they tend to turn to the Hadza. They are a throwback to a different era. And I'm not talking Prohibition or bell-bottoms. They are hunter-gatherers who spend their days hunting animals, gathering water and firewood, and picking fruits and vegetables. All that work means the Hadza walk an average of four to seven miles . . . per day.

This isn't to shame you into feeling bad about your walk to pick up groceries. Because, despite all that daily walking, the Hadza don't burn that many more calories than you or I. Hadza men burn about 2,500 calories per day and women burn 1,900 calories, even though they get more exercise in one day than the average American does in one week.

All of this is to say, while it's good to exercise (I'll outline a time-efficient, effective way later in the book), it's hard to argue that "moving more" would solve your weight gain issues. The Hadza move every single day . . . and they still aren't burning tons of calories. Because, as you'll learn later, the idea of a metabolism "boost" is very misleading. Instead, managing your weight is about managing your hunger. And that's where dieting has led you on a frustrating detour.

The more we have turned to diets to fight weight gain, the more we have paradoxically put on more pounds. In the 1950s, approximately 7 percent of men and 14 percent of women were trying to lose weight. Fast-forward to the 2000s, and that number skyrocketed to nearly 60 percent of women and 40 percent of men.[1]

And the numbers align with the changes in weight gain. In the 1960s and '70s, only 13 percent of the adult population was obese. Today, nearly 45 percent are obese and nearly 75 percent are either obese or overweight. On the surface, it would only make sense for more people to diet as more people gained weight.

But what you don't see is that the number of people dieting has been high since the 1980s, when obesity rates started to climb. Research shows that up to 40 percent of adults were trying to lose or maintain their weight throughout the '80s. That number climbed to nearly 50 percent and hovered in the 40 to 50 percent range for two decades. In other words, for thirty to forty years, half the people who need to lose weight have been trying to get healthier without success. This is backed up by research that suggests approximately 80 percent of people who lose weight will not be able to maintain it after twelve months.[2]

Clearly, the diets aren't working. And, as I've mentioned, much of the problem might be connected to the fact that when people are following extreme measures, it is harder to adopt healthier behaviors. And that means

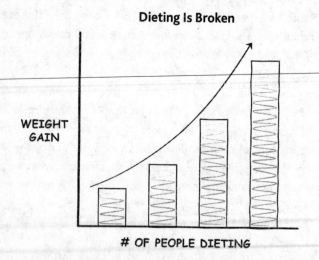

Dieting Is Broken

WEIGHT
GAIN

OF PEOPLE DIETING

the diets that are supposed to help you climb out of a hole are only digging you into a deeper ditch.

Instead of giving in to diet desperation, it helps to understand how weight loss and gain really work. Most diets hook you because they know that you want to drop pounds quickly to improve your life. But if you understand the typical rate of weight gain, it can help you understand why lightning-quick weight loss tends to backfire. Or, more specifically, why the extreme diets themselves might be an underlying *cause* of weight gain.

Most people don't pack on a ton of weight in any one given year. Instead, it's a slow burn: a couple pounds every year means we supersize ourselves decade over decade, not month over month. And that slow burn tends to be concentrated to a small window of time. Each year, people tend to do the most damage during the holiday season, or during times of extreme stress. On average, people will gain about 1 to 3 pounds during the year's final two months. In the grand scheme of things, it doesn't seem like a big deal. But, NIH-funded research suggests that weight gain during the holidays can last a lifetime. This isn't to say you can't enjoy the holidays. Instead, it shows what happens when you completely stray from normal behaviors. Most people punish themselves for enjoying Thanksgiving and Christmas by eating and drinking everything and anything. Those big meals are not the issue. It's your reaction to them that causes an abnormal shift in behavior that leads to weight gain that lasts.

If you can keep your habits more consistent and limit your enjoyment to the holidays (and not the entire month), that can make a big difference. But, that's just one piece of the puzzle. When you zoom out of those yearly trends, you see something concerning: Food has changed. Scientists of big corporations learned how to make food taste so good that it rewired your brain to desire more food, even when you'd normally feel full. The result is that you eat more than your body needs. Couple that with bigger portion sizes, and you have a multi-ingredient recipe for weight gain.

As more people gained weight, more people wanted solutions to offset the changes on the scale. I would know, because despite spending the last twenty years helping people be healthier, I found myself caught in the same dietary deadline sin.

> I've tried many diets and I always gain back the weight. And I see it coming. The plans are stressful in addition to life stress. Life gets busy and I stop doing what I need to do. But this has been different. It's easy. I don't stress. I have more energy. And I'm not waiting to end the plan because it doesn't feel like something that needs to stop
> —Andrew B.

THE CARDINAL SIN OF HEALTHY EATING

If you're not in the arena also getting your ass kicked, then I'm not interested in your opinion.
—*Dr. Brené Brown*

When I was working as a nutrition adviser to some of the biggest names in sports and entertainment–Arnold Schwarzenegger, LeBron James, Cindy Crawford, and Lindsey Vonn—I was struggling with my health more than ever. I had every competitive advantage in the world to be healthy, and I still couldn't figure it out. As much as I hated what was happening, it was clear that if I wanted to improve the physical, I needed to rethink the mental.

My problems started when I took a job that forced me to travel like never before. Every week, I'd leave my wife and two young sons and fly to Los Angeles for three days. It was one of the hardest decisions I ever made. I expected the travel to be difficult. I imagined missing my two young sons and struggling when I couldn't be there when my wife needed me most. That all played out worse than I imagined. If I could do it over, I wouldn't make the same decision again.

What I didn't anticipate was how much my health would suffer. Traveling changed the way I ate. It put me face to face with a reality I didn't fully understand before my life became a roadshow. Healthy eating becomes incredibly hard when it's not easy to cook, and you're surrounded by stress. From Tuesday to Thursday, I ordered takeout for every meal. Meals were delivered to my office in LA or my hotel room. I ate out with friends or coworkers on the nights I didn't stay in and work. And that was only part of my takeout life. Once back at home, the delivery diet continued. Every Friday night was pizza night with my family. And then Saturdays were date nights with my wife.

Add it all up, and—at a minimum—I was eating at restaurants five days per week. At my next physical, I discovered I was 5 pounds heavier. The number wasn't that big of a deal. I've never been one to stress about scale weight, but that was because I didn't need to worry about it.

I caught the fitness bug after being overweight as a child and teen, and I was one of the lucky ones; my weight hadn't changed in ten years, so seeing the new number was a bit surprising. I was less worried about my weight and more focused on what I was going to change. I thought it would be easy.

You might think the obvious answer is that I was eating takeout too often. That certainly made my life harder, and I wasn't being mindful enough of how I was eating. But many of the mistakes I was making could've been easily avoided while still having takeout. The real problems began, however, when I overreacted to the situation. My response epitomized everything that was wrong with how we approach diet, nutrition, and fitness, even though on the surface it seemed like a perfectly normal and healthy approach.

At first, I added more "extreme" behaviors I thought would work. I'd written a bestselling book about intermittent fasting, so I started there. I hadn't fasted in years (I stopped when I became a dad and wanted to eat breakfast with my son) but knew that adjustment would be easy. I returned to my old ways to shrink how much time I had to eat in a day. Instead of lunch, I used protein bars to help me get through my afternoons. And, on Sundays, I would fast until dinner and eat only one meal. I tried this for about two months and weighed myself again.

I'd gained 5 more pounds.

To be clear, fasting wasn't the problem. Intermittent fasting can help with weight loss—but it's not superior in any way to just eating on a normal schedule. But, for me, I turned a small problem into a big one. By reacting so strongly, I was overcompensating and creating unsustainable habits that were actually making my health worse, creating more anxiety, and setting myself up for bigger issues—effectively turning a Band-Aid–size issue into a bullet hole.

My weight started to become a mind game. I had put in all that effort, only for things to get worse. More concerning, it had taken me more than twelve months of travel to gain the first 5 pounds, and in less than two months, I added another 5 pounds. If this sounds familiar, it's because the path is similar for many. The harder you try, the more dramatic changes you make . . . the worse things get.

When I took a hard look at what was happening, I realized my reaction to my *perceived* screw-ups led to behaviors that only made things harder. The restrictions I created only increased the challenge of living on the road. I added stressors instead of eliminating them, which made the climb more challenging. I battled hunger more than I ever remembered, choosing meals became stressful, and I'd come back home from three days of travel and want to eat everything, knowing that Sunday was a "fasting day."

In a new environment, I also realized something I'd known existed but had never personally understood: food temptation is everywhere. Diet experts love to talk about changing what you eat but ignore that what you eat is controlled by the food around you. And that food makes your life very hard. You're told to avoid this and that. And, you probably know what to limit. But it doesn't help, does it?

IT'S TIME TO PLAY A NEW GAME

The real problem with diets—as you'll come to see—is that you've been forced to play a game you can't possibly win.

If I've heard one thing repeatedly during the years, it's this: Diets are fucking stressful. Excuse my language, but it needs to be said. (I promised my publisher I would include only one F-bomb in the book, and this was it.) Because validating your everyday reality is important if you're going to move past all your previous headaches.

When you start a diet, you sign an invisible agreement that sentences you to a life that is misaligned with your reality. It's time to acknowledge that the current recommendations for healthy eating are hard. Even harder is the work that goes into making it work for you. Most nutrition plans fail for one (or several) of the following reasons:

- Too expensive
- Too time-consuming
- Too complicated
- Too unrealistic
- Too restrictive
- Too bland
- Too boring

And when they fail, it's not like it's a slight deviation from the plan. You burn out and your brain says, "Fuck it," (I said two F-bombs, right?) and you eat everything. It's double jeopardy.

Overeating Is a Symptom

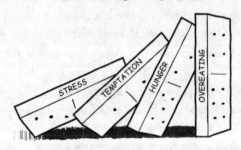

For starters, diets make eating incredibly stressful. Stress is one of the worst things for your health. And yet, these plans make you worry about *Every. Single. Thing.* you put into your mouth. When you consider that most people eat anywhere from three to five times per day, that's a lot of extra stress. If that wasn't enough, when you can't follow the plan exactly as stated—and you won't, because the rules are not realistic or conducive to your lifestyle— then you experience more stress. That leads to you overcompensating by trying to undo the behavior, which is more added stress, and then you still end up falling off the plan. Which part of this cycle is supposed to be good for you?

When this happens, diet experts will claim that you're just making excuses. And maybe you are, but—again—this is your reality. And any plan that ignores reality is a game you don't want to play. Because when you believe you must restrict, you're really playing a dangerous game with your mental health.

Researchers looked at what happens to your mental health when you go on a restrictive diet plan, such as low-carb or intermittent fasting. Now, keep in mind that these plans can be effective. But the question isn't about what can make you lose weight. It's about minimizing stress, feeling in control, and being in a good mental space so you can take care of yourself physically.

The study found that people who went on these restrictive plans had higher levels of binge eating, more food cravings, less control, more preoccupation with food, and more guilt when they gave in and enjoyed those foods.[3] In other words, restricting foods makes you crave and eat them more often, which can lay the foundation for a potential eating disorder. Binge eating or other eating disorders is not a guaranteed outcome, but believing that your body can't handle certain foods is a dangerous space.

We all live in real life, which means every meal, every day, can't be perfect. I have two kids and run three companies. Those responsibilities create real limitations on what I can and can't do to support my health. At the end of a long day, despite what I know about nutrition, it's still far easier to order takeout or microwave a meal than it is to cook something from scratch. Now, that doesn't mean you shouldn't put in extra effort to prioritize your health. It just means you need a plan that anticipates these disruptions and teaches you that you shouldn't stress those nights when you can't make the "perfect" meal. If you want to stop playing a losing game and start winning, it's time to see—once and for all—how diets are a circular pathway, and that there's a fork in the road you haven't been shown.

How Dieting Leads to Weight Gain

Diets have earned a reputation for short-term success and long-term failure. And, it's not just that they fail. It's that dieting might leave you worse than you started and more likely to gain weight in the long run. Research published in *Obesity Reviews* found that 40 percent of dieters end up heavier than before they started a diet.[4] Even more concerning is that attempts to lose weight are connected with more weight gain, even after you adjust for weight, diet, and exercise habits.

Researchers aimed to answer this exact question: Are you better off not going on a diet? Scientists at UCLA analyzed thirty-one studies that focused on long-term weight loss. The general findings were both good and bad. The good: You'll lose about 5 to 10 percent of your weight within the first six months. The bad: Up to 67 percent of people regain more weight than they lost within four to five years (and that number might be an underestimate).

Six years later, the same researchers decided to do a follow-up study, including more research to determine the weight change of non-dieters. On average, those who didn't diet gained only an average of 1.2 pounds per year.[5] In other words, when you account for the weight regain, the dieters don't end up losing much more despite their efforts. The bigger issue is that dieters don't drop many pounds, but they do gain psychological frustration from "failing" at their diet.

It's a broken feedback loop.

Each time you fail on a diet, it sets you further back. And the downward slide is exponential. The more you work on it, the more you fail and the more you feel like you're no longer in control of your eating or your health. Maybe

DIETING CIRCLE OF HELL

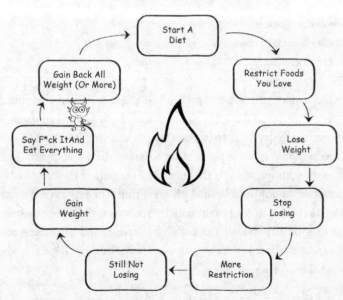

worst of all, you blame yourself and start to develop a bad relationship with your food, your body, and your life.

It's entirely possible that you would be better off if you never tried a diet rather than endless bouncing from one plan to another. Let that sink in for a moment.

If you've dieted and fallen short of your goals, you can still fix things. There are many other examples of success. One study looked at sixty years of significant weight loss and found that approximately 15 percent of people were able to maintain a weight loss of 22 pounds (or more) after three years.[6]

While it's easy to think about the 85 percent who didn't have that kind of success, there's a large enough percentage of success stories to know that long-term weight loss is possible. The key is making sure you don't fall for the traps that undercut the success of most plans. That process starts with changing your expectations on the weight-loss process.

Dad Diets Leave Obvious Clues

Have you ever noticed that all diets tend to make promises within a specific timeline?

The 4-Week Slim Down!
The 30-Day Transformation!
90 Days to a Fitter You!

On the surface, the hopeful part of you is excited about the finish line. You have a timeline and it helps you stay motivated. You tell yourself, "I can do this for ninety days!" There's something to knowing how long to measure your success. But, at some point, after so many diets and frustrations, it's worth asking this question: Is the timeline itself part of the problem?

If a diet works only for a limited period of time, the existence of a timeline is a hint that the diet will eventually let you down. Diets—no matter how similar or different—follow a curious, predictable, and disturbing pattern. You'll experience fast results and an even faster decline. It's a tragedy that occurs in three formulaic acts.

Act I: "I will succeed!"
High motivation, high compliance, high reinforcement

Time period: Weeks 0 to 3
You make changes, see changes, and believe things will work. Your weight is changing, the diet doesn't feel too stressful, and you're excited.

Act II: "I hope this keeps working!"
Moderate motivation, high compliance, low reinforcement

Time period: Weeks 4 and 5
You start to become frustrated because the weight isn't coming off as fast. You're still doing everything right, and it doesn't make sense. You have a few days where "life happens," you're stressed and want to order a burger (but you can't order the damn burger!), and for the first time, you start to hate your diet just a bit.

Act III: "I screwed it up . . . I'll start again later."
Low motivation, low compliance, negative reinforcement

Time period: Weeks 6 and 8
This diet sucks! You can't eat anything you want. You haven't had a drink in weeks. You miss carbs. You're hungry. And you gained a few pounds on the scale. *F-it! mode* is in full effect.

While the timelines might be slightly different, there's a reason why some surveys suggest that people try more than one hundred diets in their lifetime. The problem is even bigger when you consider the reverberations of your restrictions.

In general, the average person goes on a diet for six to eight weeks. When the diet increases frustration and anxiety, you quit. But it's not just that you quit; you revolt with behaviors that tend to be even worse than how you ate before you went on the diet in the first place. The average dieter follows the six to eight weeks of compliance with more than twice as much time

Why Diets Work . . . and Then Fail

TYPICAL DIET PHASES

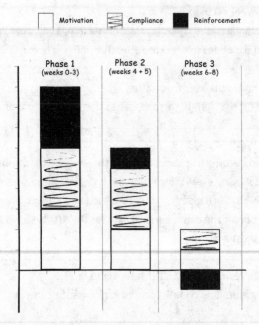

following no plan whatsoever. During that "off" period, weight tends to increase more than you lost, so the end result of all your dieting is more weight gained. It's the same phenomenon that happens during the holiday season. At some point, it's fair to ask, "What good is 10 pounds lost in six weeks if twelve weeks later you're now 15 pounds heavier?" This is the diet trade-off. You're playing short-term games with long-term losses.

The truth about diets is that they work . . . and then stop working . . . so you think you need to go on a different diet to lose weight again. All the while, each diet feels like pain by papercuts. It's rarely a big gash that makes you avoid dieting completely. You don't realize the damage until it all adds up.

For example, you might go from feeling good in your twenties to 10 pounds heavier in your thirties, and then 20 pounds overweight in your forties. It's as formulaic and predictable as the diets that took you on this journey. And because this is your reality, it's hard to ignore tantalizing headlines such as:

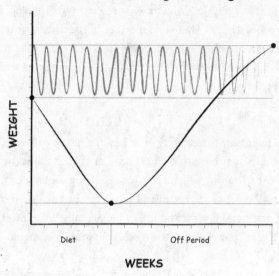

Short-Term Diets = Long-Term Weight Gain

WEIGHT

Diet | Off Period

WEEKS

7-Day Detox Plan!
Lose 70 Pounds Drinking Slimming Tea
The 28-Day Fat Torch
Fit Into Any Jeans Next Month

I didn't make these up. They are all real headlines. When you see them, your brain knows they're unrealistic, but you want to believe because you're mentally exhausted and physically struggling.

The way to break the temptation is to see that the diet is "showing its hand." This isn't their way of saying you'll get quick results; it's a confession that there is no long-term promise or commitment. Diets sell you the midpoint of the journey, not the final destination. Whether it's fair or not, it's your job to press pause before starting a relationship with someone just looking for a fling.

In order to understand the Faustian bargain, consider the following scenario: Imagine being promised $1,000 for completing a series of tasks. You're probably going to do what's needed to win the money. But what if you were told that the tasks you had to complete would lead to stress and breakdown that would cause you to quit your job, blow through your savings, and lose $10,000 during the course of the year?

Suddenly, that short-term gain doesn't seem worth it. Insert money for weight loss, and that's the trade you make with your typical diet. The problem isn't how to lose weight. There's no shortage of effective ways to help the scale go in the opposite direction. The problem is preventing the scale from bouncing back up. Or, more appropriately, it's how to improve your health without losing your mind.

Avoid the Slingshot

If you can stop falling for these empty promises, the next step is realizing that most of what these diets have sold you is BS. I'm talking about the extreme requirements to be healthy, which limit you to eating six almonds, or worrying that a small bowl of ice cream will result in obesity. When you plant these seeds of destruction, you're bound to be mentally broken to the point that you lose the willpower to eat the foods you know you should consume more often.

Diets are like a slingshot. When you restrict and remove foods, you add tension. The more you restrict, the more the tension increases. Eventually, it snaps and you fly through all your favorite restaurants, a bag of Oreos, and an ocean of margaritas with the passion of someone who just turned twenty-one. If you want to stop the rebound, start by reducing the tension you create when you start a new way of eating.

How do we remove the tension? Most people focus on the wrong question—how do I lose weight? That's why the last several decades have been highlighted by arguments about calories, hormones, and toxins. But instead of looking for a silver bullet, it's far more effective to accept and respect that weight loss is a complicated process that—for the most part—we understand. We already know the answer: creating a "negative calorie balance," or burning more calories than you store.

Now, don't confuse this for the typical "a calorie is not a calorie" conversation. What you eat matters. Certain foods help you eat less because they fill you up more or they signal reactions in your brain that don't make you crave calorie-loaded foods that tend to lead you off track. As you'll learn, the goal is *not* to restrict everything; it's just to eat more of the foods that keep you in control while still consuming enough of the foods that keep you happy.

How you go about the process is the difference breaking through and burning out. The old path makes you label foods as good or bad. And while some foods are certainly more problematic than others, forbidding these foods—at least initially—does the opposite of the intended result.

A study published in the journal *Appetite* looked at what happens when you tell people to go cold turkey on their favorite foods. This wasn't a question of calories. It was about the psychological warfare that happens when you ban foods like chocolate and baked goods. You'd think telling people to not eat certain foods would mean they wouldn't eat them. But, as any dieter knows, we want what we can't have. The researchers found that people who struggled with overeating and were told to avoid certain foods ended up eating *133 percent more calories* than those who were given no instructions whatsoever.[7]

And that was just for one day. We've seen what happens when that is applied for weeks. Again, the plans that exhaust you mentally will break you physically.

If you want to change your physiology, you have to start by changing your diet psychology. Just because you can't see what these diets are doing to your mindset doesn't make their impact any less real. It's important to know there is room for dessert and pizza. And you can map a plan so when life happens, you can order a burger and not feel like you've failed.

The other mistake is cutting too many calories too fast. This approach backs you into a corner with no escape and might increase the likelihood of weight gain and burnout. For example, let's say a diet tells you to cut all carbs. You might lose 10 pounds quickly (most of this is actually water weight), but then it'll stop entirely. What's next is proof that diets don't care about your life or your comfort. Since you can't cut any more carbs, the diet needs to start slashing calories from somewhere else. Fats are lowered. Eventually, protein—the building block of your body—is reduced too. All the while, you're becoming increasingly frustrated because you're starving and the scale isn't changing. The tension becomes unbearable.

Your body is always trying to adjust to the situation. So, taking a practical approach to learning how much you can eat and still lose is a more effective way to ensure you keep seeing progress.

Instead, it's better to discover the *most* you can eat—while still enjoying food—and still achieve your goals. This is about creating leverage. At some point, weight loss will stop. This is normal, healthy, and part of what makes it easier to maintain your new body size. But, when the stall happens, eventually you want room to make adjustments. If you start by cutting too much, you back yourself into a corner that makes it harder to accomplish long-term success.

When it comes to healthy eating, just remember you don't need black and white restrictions. And you don't need to be told something is wrong with you or your body. What you really need is an off-ramp that gives you an escape from the current diet game and a willingness to try something entirely new.

Slow and Steady Wins Big

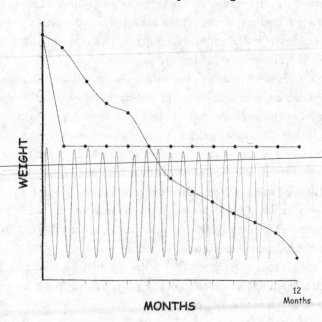

WEIGHT

MONTHS

12
Months

CHAPTER SUMMARY

- The more you diet, the more weight you tend to gain. Most people gain 1 to 3 pounds per year (you'll learn to avoid this), mostly around the holidays. But dieters also have "rebound" weight gain, in addition to holiday weight gain. Avoid the rebounds, and you're saving yourself many pounds each year.

- Don't play short-term games. Ask yourself if the plan you're following can be maintained for one year—at least. If you can't stomach the idea, it's a good sign your approach won't deliver the results you want.

- The more restrictions you make, the more tension it creates. Less friction means more consistency. Remember, people who were told to avoid all their favorite foods ate 133 percent more calories *per day*.

Chapter 3

THIS CHANGES EVERYTHING

Years ago, I hit a wall and thought, "What the hell!" Literally out of control with my weight and my body. I'm a physician, which also means I'm nerdy about all this stuff and just started reading as much as I could. It's been a frustrating couple of years. But now (in less than two months), I've lost 10 pounds. It makes sense. It's simple. You're on to something huge here and are going to change very many lives.
–Michelle C.

KNOWLEDGE IS POWER LOOKS great on a poster or as an inspirational meme. There's just one issue: The flood of information we now consume means you might have so much knowledge that it gives you less power. I'm not saying you shouldn't be informed, but I am suggesting that the volume of health information—and the difficulty distinguishing the experts from the imposters—means it's harder than ever to separate the interesting from the impactful.

In *The Death of Expertise*, scholar Tom Nichols writes that today, "We hold *all* truths to be self-evident, even the ones that aren't true. All things are knowable and every opinion on any subject is as good as any other."

Nichols's core belief is that in the internet age of endless information, knowledge isn't about knowing a lot—it's about knowing what you really need to focus on. In other words, information keeps getting in the way because we have too much of it. Some call this "the curse of knowledge." Because while it's better to be informed than ignorant, your own understanding can still create problems and blind spots. This helps explain why you've struggled to make changes that last. Not only is it harder to identify the information that will help you improve, it's harder to know when the information is most applicable to your current situation. Following advanced advice when you're still in a beginner mindset doesn't help you improve faster; it usually creates more problems, especially with something as personal and important as your health and well-being.

The "fit and healthy" often forget their own process to enlightenment. They tell you to cut out certain foods, set aside more time for exercise, have more willpower, and be motivated. The reality? No one just flips a switch and changes their habits overnight.

The healthiest people in the world don't begin with the habits that make them the healthiest people in the world. It's a gradual, flexible, and slower process than what you've been told. Most books don't retrace that journey. They just drop you at the end and expect you to skip every step along the way. It's why plans can feel impossible, and failure seems inevitable.

Diets spend too much time worrying if one food causes weight gain instead of wondering *why and how* two people can go on the same plan and one can lose weight while the other gains. Studies have compared every diet under the sun and found out that—on average—on any diet, those who are successful lose about 5 percent body fat over the course of a year. And then, because life ain't fair, most of them gain it back. That's because the strategies that help you cut calories in the short-term are a dime a dozen.

If you think you need to live in a sugar-free, gluten-free, dairy-free, artificial sweetener–free, meat-free existence, then you've been sold a lie that makes you think your body is much more fragile than it actually is. Yes, you can eventually adopt some of those lifestyle behaviors, but they are rarely the foundational first steps. You can argue about different foods for decades (just look, that's been the last fifty years of nutrition science), but it's far more important to focus on good habits, behaviors, and flexible tools.

Even before you build good habits, there's an essential step that is usually skipped. You need to develop a mindset that allows you to successfully follow the tips and plans, which means shifting self-perception. This principle of behavioral change is where all diets and workouts should start because without it, plans are most likely to fall short of their potential.

In 2017, researchers from Portugal and the UK worked with more than 2,000 dieters and focused on something that had deserved more attention for far too long: How much do your feelings about yourself on a diet impact your success with a diet?

The participants were given six different surveys that assessed aspects such as shame and guilt, social comparison, anxiety, and stress. To give you a sense of what the participants had to consider, questions included:

- *Have you ever been easily disappointed in yourself about foods you've chosen to eat?*
- *Are you ever frustrated by your unwillingness to avoid certain foods?*
- *How often are you anxious about food selections?*
- *Are you ever beaten down by self-critical thoughts?*
- *Do you believe that others think you don't do a good job of taking care of your health?*
- *Do you think your eating is inferior to others?*

On the surface, these questions might seem ridiculous. After all, who doesn't feel bad every now and then about certain food choices?

But it's worth taking a pause and really thinking about the last time you tried to eat healthier and follow a specific diet. Imagine all the things you're supposed to do, the foods you're told to eat, and the rigid plans. Now, look at the questions again and answer them from a slightly different mindset.

- *When you're on a diet, how much easier is it to feel disappointed when you didn't follow a plan perfectly?*
- *After a "bad" meal or a hard day, how much more frequently do you experience self-critical thoughts?*
- *Does it seem like others could do a better job of following the plan than yourself?*
- *Would you beat yourself up if you ate foods you were told to completely avoid?*
- *How much more did you stress about every food selection to determine if it fit the plan?*

Answering might make you uncomfortable, but exploring your reality is the exit road from the diet hamster wheel. The researchers found that variables like shame, low self-reassurance, feelings of inadequacy, and social comparison were all associated with worse weight loss outcomes and more hunger and frustration.[1]

Hundreds of studies have examined weight gain and loss, obesity, and our reactions to foods. Comparatively, very few have taken the time to understand how your self-perception and comfort on a plan either contribute to your success or are part of the reason you struggle. But, outside of dieting, we know the importance of self-perception on the ability to embrace new behaviors. And, as research continues to expand in the field of wellness, there is more evidence showing that the mental impact of diets can disrupt positive physical change.

Mental health used to be a category that only applied to serious disorders, such as depression. But today we know that your mind and body are intimately connected, and your mindset is a primary driver of your behaviors. It's never as simple as wanting to change. The best plans don't matter if the psychological strain is greater than the physical benefits. That's why the answer is clear: If you want more physical benefits, start filling your psychological cup.

The goal is to feel better about yourself. To do that, you need to be comfortable and confident. And you need to have habits and rules that support the life you want while still being healthy.

When that happens, your life will improve for the better, and you won't feel a need to go on and off different diets. You'll be at peace with the foods you eat, the plan you're on, and the person you are.

CHANGE YOUR MIND, TRANSFORM YOUR BODY

What do a 188-pound man living in South Africa and a 300-pound woman living in Memphis have in common? On paper, not much. When I met Steven and Betty, the two couldn't have been more different. And yet, both came to me from a place of deep discomfort. Steven was feeling like he was failing as a father because he didn't have the energy to run his new company

The Self-Perception Solution

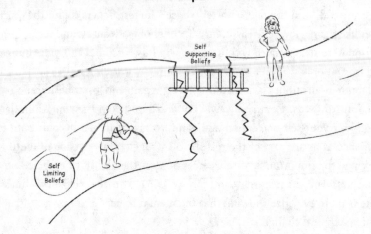

and be there for his three young kids. Betty was struggling because she worried that her weight was putting her on death's doorstep. But, more than that, she no longer liked herself because she felt like a failure.

Steven and Betty are different leaves from the same tree. When you find yourself looking for a diet, it's usually because you've had some sort of awakening. Doesn't matter if it was a doctor's visit, stepping on the scale, not fitting into clothes, or seeing an unflattering picture. Whatever the reason, you're ready for change because the pain you feel is greater than the pain it takes to change.

When I asked Steven and Betty about why they wanted to work with me, both started by painting a picture of how they wanted to feel at the end of the program. After twenty years of coaching, I've realized that people are different but the stories are similar. You probably imagine a scale with a particular number. There might be some old clothes you want to fit into again. Maybe you envision having a new sense of self. The confidence and pride. The energy you'll have, the better health, the improved life.

These are all outcomes. And it's great to picture your future self. But, having an outcome goal has little impact on the likelihood of success. Have you ever wondered why some people have more success than others? We tend to blame genetics or talk about competitive advantages such as time or money. While these can make things easier, better outcomes are not dependent on these lifestyle factors. The real key is self-perception and habit formation.

THE ULTIMATE HEALTHY HABIT

When you want to eat healthier, what's the first thing you do? Do you clean out your pantry and remove trigger foods and shop for healthier options? Maybe you search online for bestselling books, buy something from your favorite social media influencer, or ask your fit friend what they'd recommend.

Any of these could be a sensible option that helps support your health. And yet, none of them are the ideal place to start. Remember, we need to approach this in a completely different fashion than you've tried before. Throw out the cliches, zoom out, and see the bigger picture. If failures are tied to the ways that these plans break you mentally and manipulate you psychologically, then it's time to find the root cause and strengthen your foundation. After all, if you're going to be eating takeout guilt-free, well, you need to learn how to abandon the guilt.

To know where to begin your journey, it's best to understand the importance of stable foundations. Just as you would never want to fire a cannon from a canoe, starting a diet without considering your mindset and behaviors is just begging for things to fall apart sooner rather than later.

That's not to say the foods you eat, the ingredients you avoid, or the exercises you perform don't matter. It's just that if you think this is only about eating and moving, you're missing the bigger picture.

Nearly one hundred years of psychological research have suggested that if you want to accomplish a personal goal, your likelihood of success depends on your willingness to shift your identity. This sounds like a *big* change. Maybe too much for you to accomplish by reading a book. But work with me, because it's not as crazy as it sounds. The shift is about how you identify as a healthy person, not how well you've been able to find a plan that works for the goals you desire.

There's a significant difference between what you want to achieve (goals) and who you want to become (your identity). A goal is vulnerable to the endless changes in life. An identity is permanent and can weather any storm.

If you've never considered how your mindset is setting you up to fail, then what you're about to learn is going to be one of the best things you've ever done for your health.

Remember when I outlined the three acts of a diet? In the beginning, you're motivated, so you go along with the plan. Even if you're doing things you don't enjoy, your goal is strong enough that you could overcome the extreme resistance. You make it through the first week, but at some point, you know that things are going to end.

This is because two things are working against you:

1. You don't think of yourself as healthy until you reach your end goal. This mentally drains you every step of the way. Hope is tied to belief. If there's no belief, then there's no hope. And if there's no hope, the likelihood of successfully adapting to new habits is very low.
2. The juice just doesn't feel like it's worth the squeeze. Every step you take on the diet feels like a step farther away from who you really want to be. You're supposed to be feeling better, but—while the scale might change—you just don't feel comfortable with the complexity of the plan. And, in the back of your mind, you know that even if you hit your goal, it won't last because you can't keep living this way.

Now, imagine if you woke up tomorrow and believed you were a healthy person. You might not look or feel the way you want, but you didn't see that as a representation of who you are as a person. Despite not being where you want, you knew you cared about eating well and moving often.

Thinking you are something when the mirror or your habits might be telling you something else can be a difficult mental shift. It's also a very important part of success.

It helps to realize that your internal narrative plays a key role in your success in other scenarios, too. You can be a good employee before you are great at your job. You can be smart before you have the knowledge to answer complex questions. And you can be a good parent even if you haven't mastered how to raise your child.

In each of those examples, a positive self-concept plays an essential role in self-realization and actualization of an outcome. If you believe you're a terrible employee, the climb to becoming good at your job is much more difficult. Becoming healthier is very similar.

If you care about your health and are willing to prioritize it, then you need to start to believe that you are a healthy person.

Just because you haven't been given the chance to thrive in your environment, doesn't mean you're not the person you believe yourself to be. This is a big lesson from habits expert James Clear, which is outlined in his book *Atomic Habits.*

"Most people don't even consider identifying change when they set out to improve. They just think, 'I want to be skinny (outcome), and if I stick to this diet, then I'll be skinny (process).' They set goals and determine actions they should take to achieve those goals without considering the beliefs that drive their actions. They never shift the way they look at themselves, and they don't realize that their old identity can sabotage their new plans."

Clear explains that starting with outcomes-based goals (lose 5 pounds) is a recipe for failure. Instead, you need to start from a different place. First, you must start with your identity and the judgments about yourself. Just as your beliefs create hope, they also are the fuel for action. Every single healthy eating plan requires you to take action. But if you don't have the right mindset, eventually you'll run out of gas and fail.

As Clear points out, "Behavior that is incongruent with the self will not last." The biggest roadblock isn't diet or exercise—it's you. Bad diets and unrealistic workouts have supported your negative self-perception for too long. Maybe they are what planted the seeds in the first place.

Every belief is learned. And you've learned to believe some version of you not being healthy or fit. In order for anything to work—whether diet or exercise—**you need to change your identity**. The rules in this book will help you build better habits. But, in order for any of these rules to stand a chance, you need to adjust how you think about yourself.

It starts with changing your self-narrative. You might have picked up this book because you told yourself some variation of "I'm not healthy," or "I'm not in shape," or "I need to change my life." It's a negative frame that will undercut your efforts.

And yet, your actions—the commitment to buy this book—suggest something different. Reading these pages is a clear indicator that taking care of yourself is a priority. Someone who doesn't care neglects areas where they can improve. Instead of punishing yourself for not yet achieving your goals, it's important to create a positive internal narrative. Believing things like "I care about my health," "I care about my nutrition," or "I love taking care of my body," can do more for changing your outcome than any goal you set.

Changing your identity takes time, but you can shift your self-perception with a combination of beliefs, habits, and actions. The more you do something, the more it reinforces your self-belief (which is another reason why short-term plans sabotage results that last).

When you start a diet plan you know you can follow for only four or eight weeks, you build a track record of "failing" at being healthy. You're not actually a failure, but all you'll remember is starting the plan, not finishing it, or gaining back the weight. This is like jumping in the ocean with an anchor and expecting to float to the top.

Instead, it's helpful to count every win. Reading this book is one of them. Don't downplay it when doubt creeps in.

The bigger picture is seeing all your wins as evidence of the self-identity you need to develop. Each small change builds you toward a larger change. They all support the person you are—if you're willing to accept and celebrate these micro-changes, habits, and behaviors.

Changing your self-belief does not depend on achieving big goals. Remember, that's the trap. As Clear pointed out, changing your self-identity and ending self-sabotage is a two-step process.

Step 1: **Decide who you want to be.**
Step 2: **Prove it to yourself with small wins.**

When you know you care about your health, it's easy to be motivated to take healthy actions. You just have to recognize everything that counts as a healthy action rather than just counting the foods you restrict or the moments when the scale shows a lower number.

The more small, healthy actions you complete, the more you build sustainable behaviors. The more you build sustainable behaviors, the easier those behaviors become. The easier they become, the more you do them and see big results. And then, when you get those big results, they just further reinforce the self-perception you created.

THE POWER OF DISCONNECTION

There's another important trait of people who successfully lose weight and keep it off—they don't connect their value and self-worth to their weight. It's perfectly healthy to want to become healthier, lose weight, gain muscle, or have any goal related to your physical appearance. But thinking that you'll be happier because you make those changes is an illusion.

Start with Self-Perception

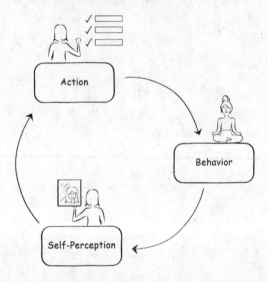

It's another health paradox, but the more you disconnect the dependency of your happiness on your appearance, the more likely you are to see the results you want.

CHAPTER SUMMARY

- Remember the big lesson about habits from James Clear: "Behavior that is incongruent with the self will not last." Start by shifting your internal narrative and giving yourself reasons to believe you're healthy. Changing behaviors is easier when you shift your mindset. You might not be at your goals yet, but that's only because you haven't found the right plan to support who you are.

- Pay attention and celebrate your small wins while not punishing yourself for the small "losses." There's no self-destruct button. You become healthier—or unhealthier—with consistent, long-term behavior. One healthy meal or workout won't lead to your desired goals, and one unhealthy meal or lazy day won't result in your body failing you.

Chapter 4

THE PARADOX OF COMFORT

WHEN I WAS FITNESS editor for *Men's Health*, I had an assignment to become super lean and achieve single-digit body fat. When I look back at what I did, the experience was one of the most eye-opening lessons, and not for the reasons you might think.

Originally, the story was going to be a step-by-step guide on How to Lose the Last 10 Pounds. But this was *Men's Health*, so the focus shifted to getting abs. If I was going to help people see their abs, then so be it. But I was hell-bent on *not* doing what had always been done. From my perspective, the world didn't need another insane workout with unrealistic time commitments. I wanted the "get abs" plan to be doable, which meant following my regular work schedule and having dessert. And, as a cheesecake lover, the combination of enjoying calorie bombs and having six-pack abs seemed almost mythical.

Since the story printed, many people ask why I made the story harder. The funny thing is, I thought I was making it easier. For one, I know I have a big sweet tooth. I was overweight my entire youth and used to need my dress pants specially tailored because my parents couldn't find slacks for someone of my short height and round width. I figured if I was going to push myself like never before, I couldn't be entirely depleted.

More important, I didn't want to create a "real person's guide to getting abs" that wasn't very realistic. I enjoy a good celeb story as much as anyone, and I've interviewed dozens of big-name stars and shared their workouts and diets. But here's the truth: It's fun to break down the routine of an actor, actress, or athlete whose primary goal and daily schedule are built around diet and exercise toward a specific goal with potentially millions of dollars on the line. But it's not exactly practical for the average person.

Real plans for real people who want to see visible results can't be too extreme or insane, because it's not realistic. You have to be in a position to graduate to that level. I can't emphasize this enough. Building momentum requires repeatable actions that you can do to gain confidence, build habits, and then progress to harder challenges that don't feel hard. I could have done two-a-day workouts or hired a personal chef and those things would've worked for me because I was in a position that they were doable. I already knew what to eat, had the discipline to navigate food temptation, and had been working out for ten years. Sure, my results probably would have been insane. But how would that help the people reading the article? It wouldn't. Not to mention, if I've learned anything, it's that most people don't need or even desire insane results. They just want to look and feel better, fit into clothes, have energy, and be comfortable in their body.

My desire to create real-life impressive results without going to unrealistic extremes created internal uncertainty. Even though it was my goal to pull it off, my closest friends knew I was unsure if I could succeed. I remember working with my diet coach, nutrition expert Alan Aragon, and he said something along the lines of, "You have some of the worst genetics I've seen." (Thanks for the confidence boost, Alan.)

Don't get me wrong, Alan was my champion and he created an amazing plan that, by the laws of science, was going to work. Still, I was skeptical about whether I could actually get great results if I didn't go to extremes and completely remove all sugar and treats.

There was something about this ambitious goal that made it seem like suffering was a necessary part of the journey. Everything in me didn't believe I would succeed, and this assignment was the ultimate test. Despite my concerns, I didn't want to back down from the challenge. The story was going to be published, and I was going to stick to my plan of doing it in a way I wouldn't lose my mind.

So, what happened?

I ate weekly desserts, and at the end of the twelve-week process, I had gone from approximately 12 percent body fat to about 7 percent. These are incredible results and surpassed even my own expectations. To be clear, that type of transformation is not "normal," and yet it happened. The fact that I achieved my goal wasn't even the best part. To my own surprise, I was able to maintain my new body size for *years*, which is far from the typical result.

As we've discussed, one of the biggest barriers to weight loss is the grind. Diets tend to be frustrating and mentally exhausting. And frustration and exhaustion lead to stress and cravings. It's a downward spiral that inevitably leads to you "cheating" on your diet, binging on foods you've missed, feeling guilty, eating more bad food, saying "F it!" and quitting the plan.

Or, you achieve your goal, think you can ease up, return to old patterns, and watch as your body shifts in ways you don't want. This leaves you feeling like the health you desire can be achieved only by following plans that can't be followed for a long period of time. It's a different experience when the plan you follow to get results is the type of plan you can stick with long-term.

Admittedly, as I followed my transformation for the magazine, I abandoned some behaviors (like drinking alcohol, something I've since added back) that weren't helping my health, but only because I was ready to do so (and not forced into it). And yet, I still left room for the things that kept me sane and enjoying the process (for me, this has always been my love of cereal, especially Frosted Flakes). And, when I had dessert (there was lots of cheesecake), I didn't punish myself with extra exercise or starve myself the following day. This was the opposite of what I had done when I lost my way during two years of travel (funny how I forgot this valuable lesson a decade later).

If you can learn what progress looks like—gradual, flexible, and filled with starts and stops—you'll find that you've probably been on the right track many times before, only to derail yourself because you were misled about the process.

NO PAIN, NO PLEASURE?

In his book *The Comfort Crisis*, author Michael Easter suggests that our modern state of extreme comfort is the cause of most of physical, mental, and emotional health crises. He doesn't just argue that we're all too comfortable, he breaks down the reasons that adding more discomfort and adversity to your life is exactly what's needed if you truly want to live a healthier, happier, and more connected life.

You might think that I would disagree, given that the cover of this book suggests that eating dessert is one of the missing ingredients of healthy living. And yet, Easter's central premise—that the extreme convenience of modern life is making us less healthy—is accurate. In his research, he found that 98 percent of people choose the easy path. For example, when an escalator is available, only 2 percent of people take the stairs. We need to embrace discomfort and even seek it in order to improve because these small challenges add up.

Using discomfort to grow and improve is often misunderstood. Just because you need to embrace discomfort, that doesn't mean you must abandon all comfort to achieve self-improvement. Most plans start with maximal pain. They ask you to jump into the deep end of the ocean before teaching you to tread water in the shallow part of the pool. When you don't know how to swim, simply being in water is uncomfortable enough. That's not to say you'll never go in the deep end. Oftentimes, you'll find out it's not as scary or bad as you thought, which is why exposing yourself to gradual discomfort is important. But getting there is a process that is usually skipped. Is it any wonder so many of us feel like we're drowning?

The idea of extreme discomfort is celebrated in all walks of life, from wellness to business. I've seen a leadership graphic that shows four overlapping circles. The first circle represents your comfort zone, which the chart suggests is bad because it's where you're safe and in control. Move out to the next circle, and you have the fear zone, followed by the learning zone, followed by the growth zone. The idea is that the farther you move from comfort, the more you find purpose and achieve your goals. It looks great on paper and seems to reflect how diets approach eating. One day you're candy and fast-food (comfort zone!), the next you're following a no-sugar, no-carb, raw, Paleo diet.

There's just one small issue. This spits into the wind of behavioral change, which suggests too much discomfort too soon will do the opposite of strengthening your mind and body; it will break you. You need a progressive approach to altering your eating habits and challenging your mind.

Most diets live in the black-and-white, and it doesn't work. Every behavior does not need to be on such an extreme scale. It's not a question of whether you always eat sugar or have none, cook every meal or eat only takeout. Yes, moderation is a helpful buzzword, but what does that really mean? In this book, a big part of learning how to grow is understanding how to *expand* your comfort zone by learning to add what is hard and balance it with what is familiar.

Discomfort is an important part of change. However, if you don't prepare your body for gradual changes, then you just set yourself up for breakdown and failure. Let's apply the discomfort principle to exercise. If you've never done a barbell squat with weight on your back, then even holding the bar can be enough to challenge you, push the limits of your comfort, and help you become stronger. This is a good starting point. However, note that this is not the same as loading up the bar with 300 pounds and telling yourself to embrace the discomfort. You'd be crushed by the weight.

That analogy sounds crazy, and yet this is the approach of far too many diet plans and some of the most popular workouts. These health plans aren't just a jump into the deep end. They are blood-soaked swims with great white sharks because too many changes are happening at once with bigger challenges than you're ready to take on. So let's reimagine the path and dose of discomfort. You don't need to be miserable all the time, nor do you need to eat only a certain way or style of food. This is based on a big misunderstanding of how we adapt to situations and create positive habits.

Most people believe that if you change what you eat, then your body will adjust and your mindset will follow. We believe that motivation flows from change. But this isn't what really happens. Instead, belief leads to action, then action leads to motivation, and that creates behaviors that last.

The saying, Where the mind goes, the body follows, is a much more accurate reflection of how lasting change occurs because behavior is driven by mindset.

If you try to build a habit without first prioritizing your mindset—or, at least, considering how your mind might react to these new changes—then you lessen the odds of success. This is known as cognitive dissonance, and it's one of the most studied psychological theories. When your actions and beliefs are not aligned, behavioral change is unlikely. And that's a primary reason why diets and fitness plans are doomed before they even begin.

Diets tend to thrive in the restriction zone, which makes it harder to accept the changes being proposed. If you've ever started a plan looking forward to the day when you can stop, have a cheat day, or "just make it through ten days of detox," then you know exactly what I'm talking about. Restrictive plans bully you into a broken relationship with food, often insisting that certain foods are bad because eating them feels good. That's messed up, and a big part of the problem.

Let's say you choose a low-carb lifestyle but you love pasta. What happens the moment you have a good Italian meal with fresh bread and an amazing plate of fettuccini? Guilt rushes in. You perceive that you're bloated. Think you can never have carbs again. And it feels like you've lost all progress. None of these are reality.

"Extreme mindsets don't work," says Dr. Danielle Belardo, a cardiologist in California. "Diets love to create black and white ideals. Low-carbers fear pasta. High-carbers fear oils and fat. Put them both on diets that avoid individual foods and—a year later—they're in the same position. No one food in one dose will cause weight gain or disease. We know that—the question is how to stop making that the focus of how people eat."

Dr. Belardo's point—no single food is the cause of health or sickness—is lost in a world of diet wars. You can eat carbs (or avoid them), but the idea of a single meal or single food making you fat and unhealthy isn't supported by one ounce of science. It's the grand illusion of nutrition.

It's time to ask an important question: Does being healthy have to come at such a high cost of living on extremes?

Dr. Belardo's approach with her patients focuses more on science-based behaviors that can help guide healthier outcomes (more plants, more fiber, less saturated fat) while obsessing less about individual foods, including occasional indulgences. If that sounds too basic, consider what happens every time you choose an extreme—the strategy most diets take: the idea that pain results in gain, and you must endure discomfort to unlock true health.

If you want to improve your health and achieve any goal, it needs to happen in your comfort zone, with steps that give you a "micro-dose" of discomfort to improve your tolerance and ability to take on behaviors that might initially feel challenging. This is where everything from takeout to dessert plays a key role in dietary success.

Finding Your Comfort Zone

Comfort is the enemy of progress.

—*P. T. Barnum (or anyone who has never successfully lost weight)*

In her research on taking risks, researcher and bestselling author Brené Brown argues that one of the worst things you can do is take risks without comfort. It might sound contradictory, but if you follow Brown's logic, it actually makes a lot of sense.

Research suggests that even when a challenge requires a lot of effort, mixing in enjoyment and feeling accomplished is a big part of success.[1] That's because accomplishment leads to more confidence, and that confidence will create consistent behaviors. Once you're consistent, you see better results and have more motivation, and that's when you can take on greater challenges (and discomfort) and make even more progress.

If consistent discomfort was the key to change, everyone would be fit because most people are miserable on diets. There's some truth to the idea that if you're too comfortable to try anything new, you don't grow. But there's a big difference between adding discomfort and completely removing comfort. People seem to think the two can't coexist, and this mentality is why diet plan after diet plan fail.

If you want to grow, you need to do things you normally wouldn't do. Also, your likelihood of success is enhanced if you take those risks in a familiar environment. The idea of "stepping outside your comfort zone" is only a half-truth: You want to step outside, as long as you still keep one foot inside. If you provide a little bit of change with a little bit of familiarity—abracadabra!—like magic, it's much easier for you to change. As time goes on, your comfort zone will change, and that's a good thing. What once seemed impossible will feel familiar, and that's how you improve.

Both feet out could mean too much stress, which results in so much fear, anxiety, and stress that new behaviors don't have room to kick in. Put more simply: It's a good thing—and ideal—if you feel a little nervous about the changes you're making. It's a bad thing if your stress and anxiety are high. In the early 1900s, psychologist Robert Yerkes built a model that explains this phenomenon: If you want great results, you want to achieve a level of "optimal arousal."

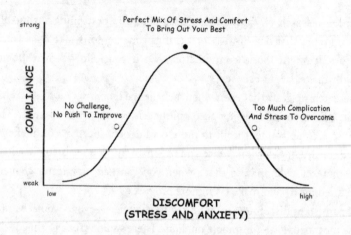

YERKES-DODSON LAW BELL CURVE
(AS APPLIED TO DIETING)

Perfect Mix Of Stress And Comfort
To Bring Out Your Best

strong

No Challenge,
No Push To Improve

Too Much Complication
And Stress To Overcome

COMPLIANCE

weak

low   high

DISCOMFORT
(STRESS AND ANXIETY)

The model shows that a little bit of stress is a good thing. But if you add too much, performance crashes. As it applies to your nutrition and eating habits, instead of extremes, you need to learn to expand your comfort zone without pushing too far or too fast. Rather than completely tossing out the old, it's more effective to introduce something new while maintaining something familiar.

Earlier in this chapter, I talked about the comfort zone graphic—the farther away you move from your comfort zone the more you improve. I'd like to suggest something different, which will illustrate a more effective way to balance comfort with discomfort.

The graphic below shows three rings, which help you identify where you are now, where you want to be, and what you want to avoid. The center ring is your comfort zone. The next ring is your improvement zone. And the final zone is the extreme zone. Both the second and third rings will provide some discomfort, but one helps you grow while the other holds you back.

Rethink Your Comfort Zone

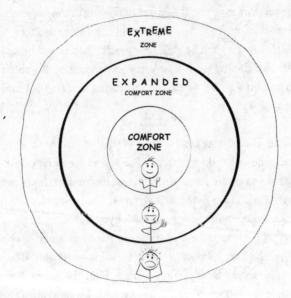

The Small Center Circle: Your Current Comfort Zone

This is where you are now. Don't think about the first circle as a representation of how you feel about your current behaviors and diet. It's not about whether you love the way you look and feel; it's about recognizing what habits feel easy. It might include things like takeout food and cake. There's a reason you eat the way you do, and trying to abandon everything you know and love won't work.

The Second Circle: Your Improvement Zone (Expanded Comfort Zone)

This is where you want to be. You want to expand your comfort zone to include some of what you know and much more of what is good for you. This happens when you use the tools you'll learn in this book. Moving to this circle doesn't mean you completely abandon the center circle. You simply add to it—and make your current comfort zone a smaller portion of how you eat and live. As you build new habits, you might find that you'll end up abandoning some behaviors completely as you add ones that make you feel better. But you don't have to drop them completely.

If the small circle is your current reality 100 percent of the time, when you expand your comfort zone you'll find yourself living in the improvement zone 60 to 80 percent of the time and in your old comfort zone 20 to 40 percent of the time. This is the goal: To gain new healthy habits and behaviors without ever fully abandoning foods that you know and enjoy. It's about enjoying takeout (but adjusting how you order) or eating dessert (but limiting how many times a week).

The Outer Circle: The Extreme Zone

This happens when you add too much change and are so far outside the first two circles that you create stress, anxiety, and discomfort. It's restriction and detoxes, shame and guilt, living on extremes. Those decisions that pull you too far outside your comfort zone will break you down.

For most people, expanding your comfort zone is a better approach for your mind, body, and lifestyle. I used to think—probably like you—that weight could be solved by flipping a switch. Find the pain point of weight gain, eliminate the pain, and you'll lose weight. I was wrong. The last fifty years of dieting have made this clear.

Successful eaters live in comfort. They have

- Better self-perception.
- The flexibility to eat without extremes.
- Less stress and guilt about their behaviors.
- Ways to control their hunger while ensuring simplicity, sustainability, and flexibility.
- The freedom to slow down and enjoy food.

Abraham Maslow's well-known "Hierarchy of Needs" shows why a fresh look at comfort can change your life for the better. Maslow proposed five different human needs: physiological needs, safety needs, love and belonging, esteem, and self-actualization.

His pyramid explains human behavior. As you satisfy your basic needs, you can move up the pyramid, take successful action, and create behaviors that benefit your well-being. But if certain foundations are not met, then it's hard to change.

Note that the second tier of the hierarchy is safety. You desire a certain level of comfort and familiarity to extend yourself and try something new. Your ability to lose weight and succeed where you've previously fallen short doesn't require you to leave your comfort zone; it depends on you learning how to increase the size of it.

Like everything in life, change happens one step at a time. But because diets prioritize rapid results over lasting transformation, you tend to skip the necessary steps that make your life easier and allow your new habits to stick because this takes time. You don't just step outside your comfort zone and magically become a new person.

In fact, growth doesn't require you to ever fully leave your comfort zone. Rather, it's about understanding how to expand the zone while never fully abandoning what you know and love.

CHAPTER SUMMARY

- Don't try to make too many changes at once. It's not necessary and will lead to premature failure.
- Discomfort is a part of growth. However, discomfort does not require you to chase extremes.
- The goal is to expand your comfort zone—not leave it completely. That means keeping things in your diet that you enjoy, which will help prevent burnout and stay consistent. And once you're consistent with new behaviors, you'll experience more success.

Chapter 5

SEEK SOLUTIONS, NOT SCAPEGOATS

DR. KEVIN HALL IS one of the most respected weight loss researchers in the world, even though the average person likely doesn't know who he is. His work has changed the way people think about weight loss, debunked flawed theories, and solved many questions about whether fat or carbs are the cause of obesity (it's neither).

Recently, he reviewed mountains of research to help explain how and why we gain weight. His big takeaway: Stop trying to blame a single food, macronutrient, and mechanism (sound familiar?). The food environment and your brain are the key characters.[1] It's not sugar, or carbs, or inflammation. They are only part of the illusion, and the reason why taking a narrow approach that focuses on a single cause will lead you right back to where you started.

Rigorous studies have searched for the best diet and come to the same conclusion. If you want to eat better, start by thinking about the plan you can follow for the longest period of time. Winning the diet game is about comfort and consistency. And you have more choice about the type of foods you can eat than you've been told.

One of the more famous weight loss studies known as DIETFITS (conducted by Christopher Gardner, another esteemed researcher), put low-carb against low-fat. It was the equivalent of the Diet Super Bowl, with a much less satisfying conclusion: the two diets tied. The low-carb group lost a little more than the low-fat group, but the amount wasn't significant, and you'd need a very powerful scale to even notice the difference.

The low-carb group lost an average of 1.08 pounds per month and the low-fat group lost an average of .92 pounds per month. To put that into perspective: low-carbers lost an average of .25 pounds a week and low-fatters lost .21 pounds per week. In accounting language, you'd call this a rounding error.

Just in case that study didn't convince you and you think low-carb is the only way to go, in 2019, the National Lipid Association reviewed more than 120 studies on low-carb and ketogenic diets and concluded, "Low-CHO [carbohydrate] and very-low-CHO diets are not superior to other dietary approaches for weight loss."

If you could speak to the top researchers who don't make money pushing a particular agenda (and yes, some scientists are tied to a belief rather than the truth), they would tell you success depends on your consistency with a plan, not the plan itself.

Scientists found this when comparing four popular diets in a study published in the *Journal of the American Medical Association*.[2] The different diets included the following:

- Low-carb/high-fat (think Atkins or Paleo)
- Balanced proteins-carbs-fats (think the Zone)
- Vegetarian, super low-fat (think Ornish)
- Weight Watchers (more food agnostic but uses points)

These diets are about as different as you can find. You're eating different foods and thus consuming completely opposite macronutrients, so you'd think one would clearly outperform the others. Yet, the best results depended less on the diet and more on how well people were to adhere to the plan.

If low-carb wasn't a good fit, then you didn't succeed. If you couldn't stick to a vegetarian plan, then you also fell short of your goals.

The research was then replicated in *The International Journal of Obesity*, this time looking at low-carb (animal-based), low-fat (vegetarian-based), and balanced (the Zone), and the amount of weight lost over a twelve-month period. Once again, the same results.[3]

Foods were secondary to fit. The researchers concluded:

Regardless of assigned diet groups, 12-month weight change was greater in the most adherent compared to the least adherent tertiles. These results suggest that strategies to increase adherence may deserve more emphasis than the specific macronutrient composition of the weight loss diet itself in supporting successful weight loss.

Not sure what any of that meant? Good, you're not alone. And this is exactly why so many people are confused about nutrition because too many brilliant scientists speak in jargon no one understands.

In simpler terms, the research provided a sigh of relief for anyone tired of feeling forced to follow a specific style of eating. That's because real-life results suggest that picking a plan you can follow for a long period of time is more likely to lead to positive results than stressing whether you should cut carbs, fat, or gluten.

Have you ever adhered long-term to a plan you hated? Me neither. Before you can start doing what's more effective, let's make sure you don't find your way back to the "ex" you're better off without.

THE GOOGLE TEST

If you've ever googled "What is the best diet?" the first page of results can have a perspective-changing impact. Once you get beyond the ads, you'll see a variety of recommendations for diets that are very different. If you read each article, you'd likely walk away incredibly frustrated and more confused than before you started. Here's a summary of the recommendations I saw while writing this book:

KETOGENIC DIETS: Remove almost all carbohydrates (you can have about 20 grams per day, or the amount of carbs in a single apple)

CARNIVORE-STYLE DIETS: Remove all fruits and vegetables

VEGAN DIETS: Remove all animal products, including things such as butter and honey (because you can't get butter without cows or honey without bees)

ELIMINATION-STYLE DIETS (LIKE THE WHOLE30): Eliminate entire food groups and ingredients, including grains, legumes, dairy, alcohol, and added and artificial sugar (you do get to add them back later)

MEDITERRANEAN- OR "THE ZONE"–STYLE DIETS: Consume a balanced mix of proteins, carbs, and fats, lots of grains and legumes, some fish and dairy, limited red meat

That's a lot of conflicting recommendations. And yet, the Google exercise provides sanity and hope in a very unexpected way. While the specific results change every year, the undeniable truth remains the same: If there were a single diet that worked for everyone, you would have heard about it by now. But the truth about dieting is right in front of us: Many diets work. And that's the point of the Google exercise. Each search result shows you a diet that is fundamentally different from the others and each has endless examples of success. Dieting is less about finding the one thing and more about understanding the principles that help drive success rather than feeling forced to eat one particular way.

And if it's not clear that the diet wars are messing with your mind and disrupting your health, consider this: If you removed all the foods that the competing popular diets tell you to avoid, what's left? Water?

It's so clear that food—in general—has been made the enemy that there are entire diets built around not eating. And you actually spend time and energy rationalizing all the reasons you'll be able to make it work:

Eating soup and juice four times per day can't be that bad?
If I never eat at restaurants again, I'll probably save money.
I don't even like food, so I'm sure fasting will be easy.

There are two ways to look at the situation: You either assume you can't win or you realize the obstacle you've been trying to avoid—"bad" food—is part of the solution to dietary freedom.

Seriously, It's Not the Carbs

The first thing clients say when I have them do the Google test is, "But I know carbs make you fat."

I say this to warn you: Don't be stubborn about a belief just because so many people say it's true. Science doesn't have feelings. It asks questions and provides answers. I also used to think carbs made people fat. I was wrong. And it's not even a question. You can cut carbs if that's your preference, but it's not necessary. I've mentioned that carbs aren't the problem, but it's worth reiterating because when doubt creeps in, cutting carbs tends to be the first reaction.

A meta-analysis (a study of studies) compared carbohydrate intake ranging anywhere from 4 percent (super low) to 45 percent (pretty high) of total calories, and fat content at 30 percent or lower in low-fat diets. Here's what the researchers found:

1. Low-fat diets were slightly more effective at lowering total cholesterol and LDL, the "bad" cholesterol that is mostly associated with clogging your arteries and contributing to cardiovascular disease.
2. Low-carb diets were more effective at increasing HDL (the healthy cholesterol that helps flush bad cholesterol out of your body and protects your heart) and decreasing triglycerides.
3. Neither diet was more effective than the other at reducing body weight, waist girth, blood pressure, glucose, and insulin levels.

The authors concluded that both low-carb and low-fat diets are viable options for reducing weight and improving metabolic risk factors. And it's not like this was a small study. It included twenty-three trials from multiple countries and totaled 2,788 participants.[4]

It's not just research that paints a clear picture. There are entire societies that prove a single food group is not the problem.

Look no further than traditional Japanese culture. Their diet is approximately 70 percent carbs and they don't have the health issues you see in the United States.

Or, read *The Blue Zones*. The popular book by Dan Buettner looks at the common traits of the areas in the world where people live the longest. The main energy sources for many of the Blue Zones are carbohydrates. Need more evidence? Many of the countries with the lowest rates of obesity consume a carb-dominant diet.

If not carbs, then maybe you're convinced sugar is the real culprit. But science would like a word with you, too. During the last twenty years, sugar consumption has dropped dramatically while obesity rates continue to climb.

Better yet, google Dr. Mark Haub and his infamous Twinkie Diet. In the name of science, Dr. Haub followed a diet of daily Twinkies (yeah, the cream-filled cakes) and lost nearly 30 pounds. Sure, it wasn't the ideal diet, and he didn't eat much else other than Twinkies, but it proved that sugar alone (even a lot of sugar, as long as you don't consume too many calories) is not preventing weight loss.

By now, I hope you're starting to see a trend with diets. Just like in a superhero movie, we're given a villain with an evil origin story who's a threat to all humanity. If we can stop the villain, we can dramatically improve your health.

The villains look different, at least on the surface.

Carbs and fats feel like polar opposites. It's a battle of which macronutrient makes you gain weight.

Diets that focus on gluten or the glycemic index turn the villain into how your body reacts to foods—there's a faulty mechanism controlling weight gain.

If you're intermittent fasting—avoiding eating at night or in the morning—then time of day is the enemy.

Detoxes and cleanses? They focus on toxins and inflammation, two things that sound terrible but are very much misunderstood. For example, if you removed all inflammation from your body, you'd probably become very sick. Inflammation is a key ingredient in how we react and respond to stress and illness.

The list goes on and on. You can paint the experience a million different colors: Diets ultimately rely on the same trick.

- When you remove carbs, you eat fewer calories and eat less.
- When you fast, you eat fewer calories and eat less.
- When you restrict gluten or dairy, you eat fewer calories and eat less.
- When you go Paleo, you cut out other food groups and eat less.

The Real Reason People Lose Weight

ALL DIETS RELY ON THE SAME TRICK

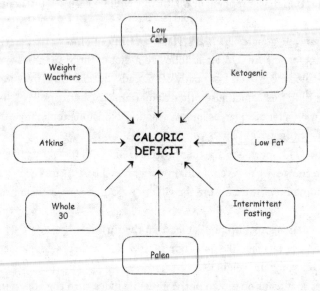

Everything is a manipulation of energy balance. That's not to say other mechanisms aren't involved in weight loss. In fact, Dr. Kevin Hall (the brilliant researcher mentioned at the start of this chapter) suggests that the brain and hormones play a big part in determining your weight. But diets are leaving out information that explains why—even after you lose weight—you gain it all back.

It's much easier to sell the dream of weight loss than the reality of how your body really works. When a plan stops working, it's easy to suggest another supplement, superfood, or detox. But, none are the answer you seek. These roads only make it easier to suggest you're not committed, lack willpower, or—worst of all—infer that you have a "broken" body.

If you've ever felt that way, I'm sorry. That's BS.

You're not broken. Your weight is not a reflection of you. And it's likely not an issue of commitment or willpower. No matter what you've been told, there is a better way.

MOVE BOULDERS, NOT PEBBLES

How much do you focus on adding superfoods to your diet? What about stressing over how long you should fast between meals? Do you choose your workouts by obsessing over the "best" exercises?

Those details all count for something, but they require a lot of energy for very little reward. They say the devil is in the details, but in fitness and nutrition, sometimes the details act like the devil. They trick you into focusing (and stressing) over minor decisions that don't lead to major results.

If you want to change for the better, you can't stress every decision. Remember, the "Google test" helps you understand that many plans work. The piece that is missing—the one thing that Google can't answer—is determining what will work for you, based on your preferences and lifestyle.

If you love carbs, don't build your diet around keto. If you barely have time for friends and family, don't start with a program that requires six days per week of exercise. That's not to say those are bad plans. It's also not to say you won't end up following a plan like that one day. It does mean that if you want to get to a better tomorrow, you need a plan that supports a better today. That means focusing on behaviors that are easy for you to follow and that make a big difference for your health. These are the boulders.

Most of the details you're told to worry about are pebbles.

- If a diet makes you stress the little things, then it's missing the big picture.
- If you need to worry about a specific hour to eat? It's a problem.
- Not sure if you can add a little creamer to your coffee? It's a problem.
- Afraid to eat a sandwich because it has bread? Well, that's no good.
- Think drinking one diet soda will cause cancer? Yep, still a problem.

In life, there are big problems and little problems. With health, too often, people turn little problems into big problems, and then every problem feels huge and you're swallowed by it all because it feels overwhelming.

You can't turn off the volume of the information, but you can learn to block out the noise. Here's what really matters if you want to see success:

STAY NOURISHED: Eat more nutritious foods—whether processed or unprocessed—that keep you full, satisfied, and energized.

REMAIN SANE: Leave room for some of the foods you love because restriction leads to a lack of consistency.

AVOID GUILT: Stress and anxiety will break even the healthiest plan. If a plan makes you sorry about everything you eat, then guilt will make it impossible for you to create good habits.

These are the components of a solid foundation. You'll learn how to stay nourished, sane, and avoid guilt throughout the rest of the book. That means you don't need to stress how many meals to eat in a day, the exact timing of those meals, or whether a little bit of creamer or diet soda will ruin it all.

MAKE IT HARD TO FAIL

One of the most underrated resources for winning against weight loss is the National Weight Control Registry (NWCR). It doesn't provide a specific diet or workout. Instead, the NWCR spends its time learning from more than 10,000 people who have lost weight—and kept it off—for years. It's the holy grail, the Loch Ness monster, and the needle in a haystack all wrapped in one. Why spend time searching for a diet that might work for you when you can find the lessons that work for people across many diets?

The first thing you'll realize from the data at NWCR is that their recommendations are rarely the tips you see in popular diet books. They're almost too boring, which is why you don't hear about this information more often. If you're trying to get people to start a new behavior, basic principles rarely work to initiate action.

If I were to try and convince you to eat more fruit or protein as a means of losing weight, the likelihood of acceptance is low. But, if I were to tell you to try "intermittent fasting," then the initial rate of adherence is high. The end goal is the same (eat less food), but the novelty and complication of fasting directly impacts your willingness to engage (even if it's not desirable or sustainable).

European researchers examined this phenomenon by using fMRI to see how your brain reacts to new information. Any time you're presented with something new, the parts of your brain (known as the substantia nigra/ventral segmental area or SN/VTA) lights up.[5] This is important because that pathway triggers dopamine.

You might remember dopamine from your high school education. It's the feel-good neurotransmitter. As it applies to nutrition and fitness, a shot of dopamine increases motivation, drive, and focus. It's why it's almost impossible to resist the new ideas that might make you better, no matter how crazy those new ideas might sound. It's not just that you're motivated; your brain is wired to associate novelty with reward.

One of the lead researchers of novelty research stated:

When we see something new, we see it has a potential for rewarding us in some way. This potential that lies in new things motivates us to explore our environment for rewards. The brain learns that the stimulus, once familiar, has no reward associated with it and so it loses its potential. For this reason, only completely new objects activate the midbrain area and increase our levels of dopamine.[6]

Translation: Your brain is likely to skip over information that feels like common sense and believe that something new is more likely to lead to reward. Which is why the data from the NWCR is so important. It helps to pay more attention to the data because it provides clues for how to break the vicious cycle of dieting. And yet, your brain isn't excited by the info because it seems too boring.

It helps explain why bold claims that focus on "cutting-edge ideas" and extreme behaviors tend to go viral and get headlines (I'm looking at you, Celery Juice Diet).

The "boring" strategies are what scientists call valid and reliable. They don't get the headlines, but they are the gold standard for making claims with more certainty. These are the ideas that are most likely to lead to predictable outcomes. If you wanted to make a good investment that pays off, then you rely on valid and reliable research.

But—and it's a big but—in order to establish reliability and validity, you need to test . . . and test . . . and test, again and again. The mere process of creating certainty removes the novelty. So, what works best is also what is least exciting or motivating. The question you need to ask yourself is simple: After so many years of uncertainty, are you willing to choose the boring recommendations instead of the bold?

Doing so might make all the difference. If you're still uncertain, know there are many advantages to boring recommendations.

New, bold ideas are rigid and difficult to follow. They break easily. It's why every extreme plan falls apart with the least amount of friction. The examples are endless. A small amount of carbs take you out of ketosis. Eating solid foods ruins your detox. Consuming any food ends your fast.

It's far better to have a flexible structure that you can bend to your will without it ever snapping. What if you could bend a plan to your lifestyle rather than having a plan bend your life? The more comfort you experience on a diet, the more likely you are to keep the weight off. If you recall, only about 10 to 20 percent of people who lose weight are able to keep it off.

And yet, a study in the journal *Obesity* found that dieters with high adherence were much more successful more than two years after they started the plan. Instead of the usual grim stats, people with high adherence regained only 50 percent of the weight they lost, which is a big difference. In this particular research, people with low adherence regained 99 percent of the weight they lost.[7]

And that's what makes the NWCR so compelling. They have amazing success by doing boring things incredibly well. Here are some of the common traits of people who successfully master long-term weight loss:

- Eating carbs
- Enjoying breakfast
- Avoiding extreme restrictions and gimmicks
- Limiting but not completely removing ultra-processed foods
- Prioritizing movement

There are a few more habits—such as weekly weigh-ins—but 80 percent of the habits are based on mastering simple concepts. It's not about the extremes. It's about the things you can easily repeat that keep you on-track and make it almost impossible to get off track.

If you analyze those traits and search for a common thread, it's that every primary decision prioritizes flexibility and expands the comfort zone without going to extremes.

When you look at it that way, it's easy to ask, "What if good nutrition isn't about getting on or off a style of eating?"

My hope for you is that the results of the NWCR inspire a, "Well, look at that!" moment. You have the power to change the likelihood of success by choosing to follow a more practical plan. Success depends on having a plan that fits your lifestyle preferences. If you're ready to live the healthier life you deserve, then it's time to open the third door.

THE THIRD DOOR

Life, business, success . . . it's just like a nightclub. There are always three ways in.

Those are the words of Alex Banayan, author of *The Third Door*. In the bestselling book, Banayan interviewed many of the most successful people in the world and determined that the common denominator was the ability to find a non-traditional path that most people overlook. Banayan outlines the three pathways you can choose, which include the following:

THE MAIN ENTRANCE: where 99 percent of people wait in line, hoping to get in.
THE VIP ENTRANCE: where the billionaires and celebrities slip through.
THE THIRD DOOR: "It's the entrance where you have to jump out of line, run down the alley, bang on the door a hundred times, crack open the window, sneak through the kitchen—there's always a way."

Dieting is much the same. If you were to apply Banayan's logic to nutrition, it would look something like this:

THE MAIN ENTRANCE: You've been there before. It looks like extreme restriction, unrealistic plans, and very little flexibility. It's the crash-dieting techniques that help you lose weight fast—and then gain it all back. It's a roller coaster, a yo-yo, and a path that—in the long run—leads to failure for the vast majority of people.

THE VIP ENTRANCE: Some people have competitive advantages. It's just the way of life. Think unlimited budget for food. Expensive personal trainers. And a schedule that helps reduce the real-life stressors, such as a lack of time.

THE THIRD DOOR: A hybrid approach that turns everything you thought was important on its head. It's a side door that focuses on the lessons of successful dieters, avoids the mistakes of failed diets, and adds a bit of novelty— restaurants and processed foods are not completely restricted.

It's an approach built on adding sustainable methods of eating nutritious foods that don't take a lot of time and budget, while providing the freedom to eat foods that are both familiar and enjoyable. This means leveraging "the big three" pillars of healthy eating. That includes consume foods that (1) nourish your body, (2) protect your sanity, and (3) avoid guilt.

Opening the third door means trading the smoke and mirrors of immediate results for something that seems almost too good to be true. A practical plan that allows you to eat more of the foods you love while still losing weight. It's not a gimmick. It's just the opposite. It's the first plan that is honest about how quickly you can realistically lose weight, how your metabolism *really* works, and why more diet breaks and a little bit of imperfection is exactly what you need to end the vicious cycle of dieting.

THE FORK IN THE ROAD

You now know that you need to build a new self-identity, expand your comfort zone, and find the third door. Those three changes can lead to dramatic health improvements. However, it only makes a difference if you build your foundation on those principles. Otherwise, you'll still be at the mercy of the dieting hamster wheel.

If you choose the road less traveled, then there's one more step that will ensure you never return to the old game: You need to know how to avoid the tension, stress, and frustration that typically derail a good plan. The next section of the book will cover how to develop the right mindset, outline the foods that you need to limit the most, and help you understand the best way to achieve weight loss that lasts. If you feel you have a strong grasp on all of those concepts, then feel free to skip to section three and dive into the tools and eating plans.

But, a word of caution: I've worked with many people who think they know the enemy, only to be ambushed by something they never expected. In the next section, you'll learn about the mental, environmental, and physical barriers that you'll face because you don't live in a controlled environment. When real life happens, you need to know what to expect so you can easily navigate the situation. Life is filled with "trap doors," but if you know where they are located, then it's much easier to make sure you don't fall.

CHAPTER SUMMARY

- There is no single best diet. I repeat: Many diets work. Adherence is what allows a diet to deliver results.
- Adherence is hard if you hate what you're eating, are constantly stressed or anxious, or don't believe you have flexibility to be adaptable. Diets, like people, can't be fragile, or else they break. Your plan should feel resilient.
- Carbs don't make you fat. Neither does the timing of your meals, gluten, or the glycemic index. Either you eat too much or you don't. Having a plan that helps you stay full without breaking your will (see the big three) is what makes this doable. Embrace the big three: consume foods that nourish your body, protect your sanity, and avoid guilt.

PART 2

IN CONTROL

Chapter 6

NOTE FROM YOUR FUTURE SELF

Trying to be too perfect is a huge problem for people in diet world.
—*Dr. Yoni Freedhoff*

CINDY CRAWFORD'S DIET WOULD probably blow your mind. That was the first thing I thought when I sat in her kitchen and watched her make, bake, and eat an incredible rhubarb pie filled with a whole lot of deliciousness. I've interviewed celebrities and athletes for fifteen years, and Crawford's style of eating was refreshing and gave me hope for the future.

Many celebs are frequently going on and off diets. There's nothing sustainable about it. They have to look a certain way, and to do so, they'll go to extremes . . . until it breaks them. But, we'll celebrate the dramatic change or beautiful appearance, and overlook what it took to get there. And yet, here was Crawford, the supermodel of all supermodels, now in her fifties, talking about her love of baking pies with her children, eating them, and enjoying every bit of each bite. When I asked her about her approach, her philosophy surpassed that of many brilliant dietitians. "I try to be 80 percent good, 80 percent of the time."

In saying so little she established so much about why her approach works. She didn't say she could eat whatever she wants. Crawford has a simple, flexible way of thinking about food. She limits ultra-processed, packaged foods. She makes sure she has a filling breakfast to limit cravings and enjoys protein at her meals. She has small snacks when she's hungry. But it's the dessert part that stuck out. Because it's not just what she's figured out. It's what she's passing on to her family, including her daughter, Kaia, who is also a successful model.

"The idea that dessert is unhealthy is an unhealthy mindset. I don't want to fall for that trap, and I don't want her to think that's necessary. So whether it's baking pies or having a small piece of chocolate after lunch, it's important to normalize what we've been taught to think is bad. But it's the extreme perfection that is really the problem."

In a world of short-term fallacies, Crawford played the ultimate long-term game, and she looks as good as ever, proving that letting go of perfection is a much healthier—and more fun—way to eat well. While most people over-analyze everything they eat, Crawford's ability to not overthink makes the biggest difference because she avoids the guilt and shame, and then doesn't do anything special to adjust for her normal indulgences. They are all part of the plan.

THE ART AND SCIENCE OF HEALTHY EATING

In *The Subtle Art of Not Giving a F*ck*, bestselling author Mark Manson argues that the "cult of positivity" does harm to your self-development. Manson argues that a path of selective indifference is the true path to happiness, calmness, and feeling more in control. In a nutshell, he states, "Not giving a fuck does not mean being indifferent; it means being comfortable with being different." (Okay, last F-bomb. I promise.)

His point is you can't care about everything, which is exactly what Crawford discovered on her own journey to health. Stressing every decision or calorie is a path to burnout and self-destruction. But you should care about some things. This is the ultimate revelation with healthy eating, and why healthy eating is different than dieting.

Diets are built on a strict set of rules. Healthy eating is about embracing all foods and making good decisions often—but not always. You can't care about every morsel of food you put into your mouth. It's doing far more harm than good.

I first realized this when helping a client named Donna, a woman in her mid-forties who had struggled with her weight for the previous fifteen years. When we met, she was at the point of giving up on her body. She was tired of trying to add vegetables to her diet and didn't see the point of exercising when the scale didn't move. She figured she might as well just eat whatever she wanted and stop putting in so much effort.

One day, I told her I wanted her to *get comfortable with falling off the wagon—as long as she never abandoned the wagon.* Donna thought I was insane (even I wasn't sure if I made sense), but six months later—and twenty pounds down—she would tell me it was the moment that changed everything. Because it helped her see that she could eat some of the foods she loved and still see results. Before, it was all or nothing. Each time she had dessert, she felt she "lost" and followed up with many other unhealthy meals, instead of realizing that just because something didn't have nutritional value didn't mean it was unhealthy and unacceptable.

Your expectation about what it takes to be healthy isn't aligned with reality. The occasional treat, dessert, or enjoyable meal is not what stops progress. It's when you go into a guilt cycle, followed by behaviors of complete restriction or no regard for your health whatsoever, that things fall apart.

Great health is accomplished by being "good enough." When I think about making healthy decisions, I assume that approximately 25 percent of my days are going to be a struggle, 50 percent of my days are nothing special (but lead to small positive changes), and 25 percent of my days I'll feel like I'm doing great.

On paper, this doesn't look like a recipe for success, but the math works in your favor. The crappy weeks are crappy, but they are better than nothing. The 50 percent weeks are when you're making those small incremental changes that are the foundation of success in anything. And the 25 percent of the time when you are better than average gives you that extra boost and motivation.

Add it all up, and you see that even if 75 percent of the time you won't feel like you're doing enough, you're still getting better because you didn't completely stop trying. Most importantly, it takes the pressure off so many different meals that typically are the first domino that causes your plans to fall apart. Part of doing things differently is learning a new style of eating. The other part is finally recognizing how prior methods would leave you broken.

THE STRESS TEST

"When was the last time you didn't worry about what you ate?"

I've asked this question to many clients, and it's the moment that usually helps them understand that their relationship with food is broken and doing far more harm than they ever realized.

Eating is necessary. And it's meant to be enjoyed.

And yet, food is stress quicksand. The more you fight your anxiety, the more you get overwhelmed by it. You worry about which foods are acceptable to eat. You worry if you're eating too much—or not enough of the right foods—and you tend to worry that you're doing damage when you eat something unhealthy. And even if you don't worry, you definitely feel guilty.

Food anxiety follows you everywhere. Before meals, during meals, and after meals. This is a big reason you struggle to find a plan that works and you end up settling for quick fixes. You can only handle so much stress before it takes over your body and affects everything from your decision-making to the hormones that help you function your best. When you're overstressed, you have less willpower and are more likely to make decisions you want to avoid. You start to crave foods you want to limit, and it's easier to gain weight and harder to burn fat.

To top it off, stress makes it harder to sleep, which only means your decision-making gets worse, your hormones break down more, your cravings go through the roof, and your focus and motivation are tapped. Stress is a part of life, but it doesn't have to be a part of eating. If you can reduce how much you worry about food, you can change your relationship with food, be in control more often, eat, and enjoy.

You might be wondering where you draw the line between giving yourself grace and challenging your comfort enough to grow and improve. The answer is the inverse of what you've been told before. If the old way was to be perfect all the time, then the new way is to never be completely imperfect.

How Stress Leads to Overeating

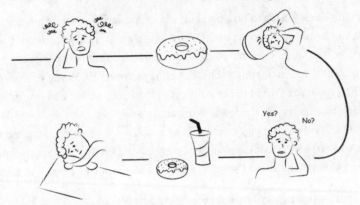

Avoid Zero Percent Weeks

In *The Subtle Art*, Manson shares, "This book will help you think a little bit more clearly about what you're choosing to find important in life and what you're choosing to find unimportant." I hope this book does the same for eating. What's unimportant is being perfect.

The problems start when your frustration takes you down to zero percent. On some level, you need to realize that minimal efforts done over time can help you build consistent habits. Like building a muscle, you just need more reps. Those consistent habits help change behaviors. Those changes will lead to positive results. When that happens without having to sacrifice everything, you build confidence and start removing more of what doesn't serve you, which is when you maximize results. It's all a gradual process that begins when you decide to not quit on your health.

If 75 percent of the time you were doing something to be healthy, 25 percent of the time you're doing almost everything, and you have no weeks with zero percent, then you would be 110 percent healthier several months later. Learning to embrace "good enough" is the mindset that matters.

Compliance was probably about 85 percent for last week. I ate too much over the weekend. But, no guilt and just went back to normal the next day. I've never done that before. The crazy part? I lost weight! To lose weight without feeling like I am trying to lose weight is pretty cool
—*Laura W.*

Health doesn't have to be a bargain, where you sacrifice everything. Even when you bend the rules, it's not the end of the world. And knowing it's not the end of the world prevents things from spiraling. That is the secret to being in control and increasing your comfort. If you never think you've screwed up, then you don't give in to the guilt cycle of anxiety, stress, and overeating or reach more often for the foods you want to avoid.

Often, it's not what you eat that's the problem. It's how you respond to what you eat, which leads you to frequently eat the foods you want to limit. Instead of worrying about the scale, start by asking yourself these questions:

How much stress and anxiety does your diet cause?
How much do you worry about food?
How much do you count the days until you can be "off" the diet?
Is the way you're eating really making your life better?

Answering these questions will help walk you away from plans that you won't be able to follow and move toward a more sustainable, effective approach.

The Unhealthy Health Obsession

Brownies made from black beans are not brownies. Pizza made on a "crust" of eggplant is not pizza. And cookies with raisins are not cookies. (Okay, maybe they are, but few things are worse than thinking you're biting into a chocolate chip cookie only to discover the "chips" are really raisins.)

The idea that all foods need to have nutritional benefits has made you lose your mind and debate things that should never be debated. If you want to make black bean "brownies," then please do so. Same goes for the flourless pizza. There's no problem modifying ingredients in treats to make them healthier (you'll find examples in the recipes, which start on page 173).

The problem is how we talk about treats, indulgences, and high-calorie foods. The question isn't about what happens when you swap—it's about what happens when you don't, and the amount of guilt it creates. It's dangerous and unhealthy to obsess about everything you eat. Counting calories can be an effective tool, but for many people, constantly worrying about every single calorie or macronutrient becomes a burden that does far more harm than good.

Your health is the single most important investment you can make. Eating plays a big role in making sure that investment pays off in the long run. None of this means you need to trick yourself into believing beans are brownies or think a single meal or dessert will make you fat. If this describes how you feel when you order takeout, eat dessert, or have alcohol, consider this a warning.

Simple math shows how this quickly becomes a problem. Three meals a day equal twenty-one extra stressors per week. Go on a diet for a month and you're adding stress nearly one hundred more times—on top of the other life stressors you already manage. This is too much. The internal battle you're waging is making it harder to lose weight and be healthier than any genetic limitation you might have.

Researchers at the University of California found that women had more perceived stress when they followed a diet for three weeks. This might not seem like a big deal, but the increase in stress can turn your body against you. In the study, the dieters were 66 percent more likely to have increased cortisol,[1] a hormone your body releases when you're stressed. Cortisol is connected to many frustrating conditions, and one of them is—you guessed it—weight gain.

Stress is the enemy of health and weight loss. If stress happens infrequently, then no problem. Your body can handle stress. In fact, it's built for it. If it happens a lot, that's a different story. Stress creates a tipping point, and your hormones shift. You won't feel it directly, but your body will let you know something has changed. The more stress you add to your life, the more you have to double or triple your efforts to be healthier.

Even the slightest decision can be a trigger. Let's say you want a brownie. You feel guilty, but you make them and eat a few—but you don't really enjoy the process. Next thing you know, you feel like a failure. You start stressing about the calories and sugar you ate. You're mad at yourself for not being stronger. And, because you already feel like you blew it, you go ahead and have a few more brownies.

The calories you consumed might be more than what you want in that moment, but one meal is just one meal. It's easy to get lost in that moment. But, in the context of a week or month, it's a rounding error that would have little to no impact on your health. If you just enjoyed and returned to your normal eating, your body wouldn't notice, and your mind would be satisfied. But what matters much more is what's happening between your ears. In the scenario above, the brownies aren't the main problem. It's how you quickly added up too many anxiety points. And those stressors start altering the way your body normally functions.

Usually, when you eat, your body receives fullness signals. But, when you're too stressed, it's harder for you to feel full. The anxiety can also impact your sleep, which can make you ravenous and craving every single food you want to limit. Meanwhile, the stress is making it harder to recover, have mental clarity, exercise, and do your job.

What happens when you can't exercise, you're overtired, and you're stressed by work? We've all been there. You get hungry and crave all the foods that are the furthest thing from healthy. In the current diet environment, you don't stand a chance. The "don't eat this and don't eat that" mentality pushes you toward stress when we live in an environment where delicious food is more available than ever.

Meal delivery apps aren't billion-dollar companies because they have cool names. You're going to eat takeout (we all do!). You need a plan that accepts your reality—not one that acts like you're a robot without temptation, a job, or nights where laziness forbids you from cooking a healthy meal.

Your reality can be a part of a healthy existence; you don't always have to eat foods that get a gold star from a nutritionist. However, it's important that you feel good about your decisions and not let stress follow every food decision.

How to Embrace Guilt-Free Eating

The more shame and guilt you feel, the more likely you are to overeat, struggle with hunger, and gain weight.

THE STRESS-EATING CYCLE

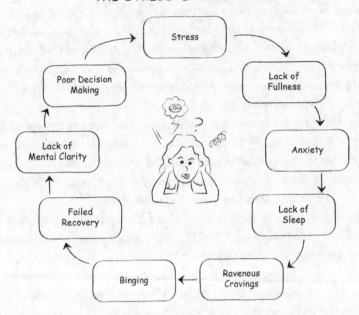

But, what about those who don't experience those emotions?

People who don't worry about everything they put in their mouth—and even feel good when they eat less-than-healthy foods or are not at an ideal weight—tend to have better outcomes, less stress, and are more likely to stick a plan. This makes perfect sense when you consider everything you've already learned about self-perception, the diet slingshot, and the ways stress and anxiety from well-intended diets send you on a tailspin.

Feeling better about your health isn't just about the foods you eat, it's about how you feel when you eat healthy *and* unhealthy meals. In fact, when you stop viewing everything as healthy or unhealthy, it can go a long way toward helping you feel fuller, which is a key ingredient to managing hunger, a big problem for most people who change their diet. That's because when you hear the word "healthy" your brain processes it as "unfulfilling." In one study, people were given a "healthy" chocolate bar, a "tasty" chocolate bar, or no food at all. Even though both bars were exactly the same, those who had the "healthy" bar felt hungrier than subjects who ate the tasty bar and those who ate nothing at all.[2]

Now, in real life, you can't trick yourself into what you're eating. Not to mention, when you want to eat healthier, you're naturally going to go for the foods that are marketed as being better for you. And when you do—whether they are actually good or not—you're likely to feel hungrier and then desire more food. This, along with many other reasons we've covered, is why it's not only important, but also necessary, to retrain the way you think of food and embrace a different style of eating.

Yes, there are limits on what you can eat. And yes, you'll want to eat those healthier foods, which can take time and requires some adjustment. But, the biggest adjustment needed is how you feel about yourself and how you rate and compare foods. Because your perception about foods can influence the chemical reactions occurring in your body.

Research suggests that the perception of fullness can cause your body to release a hormone called GLP-1, which is a powerful appetite suppressant.[3] GLP-1 drugs are now being targeted by pharma companies as the gold standard in creating long-term weight loss, and the results are unlike anything we've seen before. But, these drugs are still new and very expensive. If you can flip the switch in your brain about how you perceive food, then you can potentially help yourself get some of the benefits without paying for the medication

This might feel like a massive shift. However, you're more prepared than you think. To make the jump, you need to think less about the health values of different foods, embrace your imperfections, and build grit.

GRAY THINKERS LOSE WEIGHT

The ability to avoid black and white thinking could be the difference between leaving the dieting hamster wheel or continuing to run in circles. People who lose weight and keep it off are great at avoiding dichotomous thinking.[4] In other words, if you want a better relationship with food (and some impressive results) you can't be thinking every food, ingredient, or meal is an all-or-nothing decision, healthy or unhealthy, good or bad.

Those who change their outcomes don't focus on being perfect with every meal. They don't react to small changes on the scale. And they are able to see that even the smallest victory—such as including protein in a meal—is part of what it takes to be healthier.

I said it earlier in the chapter about behavioral change, and it's important to remember now, that winners celebrate every success. Those who struggle dwell on every hypothetical failure. But you can't build a successful plan on top of stress. It's like building a home on a faulty foundation. You can have the best materials (best foods), but if there's no foundation that can weather the storm (real life), then everything crumbles. To reduce stress, you need to know that no one single food or single meal ruins your health. In other words, nothing is off limits.

Difficult Dieting Past = Happier, Healthier Future

One of the most common errors is giving into the temptation for a bright, shiny new diet or workout that promises better, faster results. Research from fifty years ago shows why it's a trap that's hard to resist.

In 1972, an experiment on children laid the foundation for decades of psychological manipulation that is used by marketers to this very day. The study occurred at Stanford University, where lead researcher Walter Mischel was interested in learning about delayed gratification. In particular, he wanted to understand what it would take to reject an initial reward and wait a longer period of time for a greater prize.

At the time, it was one of the most pivotal studies in judgment, decision making, and long-term behaviors. The findings have been picked apart over the past few decades, and it has a few flaws. But, when it comes to unlocking better health, one of the core concepts of the research can help you avoid many common missteps and frustrations.

In the experiment, children sat in an empty room where researchers had placed a desired treat (marshmallows) on a table and offered a simple proposition: You can have the treat right now or wait for fifteen minutes and get double the deliciousness. The researchers then left the children alone.

The researchers originally believed that the bigger reward (more marshmallows!) would be enough to delay gratification. But once the experiment began, most kids couldn't wait. The temptation of the marshmallow was just too much to overcome. The research helped define principles of focus and action. Specifically, this study helped clarify that it's very hard to wait for a bigger prize if you can't distract yourself from the seemingly easier win. When children would focus on getting more marshmallows it did the opposite of what the researchers thought—it made them want the quick solution even more.

Waiting for a better outcome wasn't a matter of thinking about a greater reward. It was dependent on whether you could distract yourself from gratification entirely. Even though we become smarter as we age, the psychology of gratification is surprisingly similar to your childlike instincts. When you want something, it triggers a form of desperation that narrows your focus and doesn't allow you to think quite as clearly. This happens all too often with dieting. Opting for a quick win like "lose five pounds in five days" is just a way to ensure that you're going to lose out on the greater reward and repeatedly be frustrated with your experiences and results.

Knowing that you want to distract yourself from short-term goals doesn't make it any easier to do so. In fact, it can make it even harder. And that's what fascinated researcher Angela Duckworth, the author of *Grit*.

Duckworth was less interested in *if* you could distract yourself from the prize and more curious about how you develop focus and persistence. Her research found that you need to develop two qualities: motivation and volition. And it's a lock and key relationship. If you don't possess both, then you're not likely to succeed.

Most of us don't have an issue with motivation. It's not a problem of wanting to become healthier. It's the volition—or self-control and willpower—to stay the course when times are hard, stress is overwhelming, and the idea of a pint of ice cream is just too much to resist. When you have both of those, it becomes easier to stay the course. But there's one other missing piece that truly determines the highest likelihood of success—*grit*.

Grit is the X-factor that helps you stay on-track during a long-term goal, such as lifelong health. It's a dedication to a particular mission, such as being able to live the life you want. When you consider the importance of changing your self-narrative, you can see how well these puzzle pieces fit together.

If you believe you're a healthy person, it's easy to attach a stronger purpose to your goal, which means you can develop the grit you need to succeed.

So where do you start with grit? Understand that your past failures are *not* failures. Rather, they are part of the journey of learning and mastery. Duckworth's research probably sounds similar to advice you received as a child: mistakes are your best teacher. And, if you make mistakes and learn from them—rather than punish yourself—then you can build grit that will serve you in the long-run. This is invaluable when it comes to dieting, especially if you stop feeling guilty for everything you eat and enjoy.

It's time to change your perspective on your previous attempts to eat healthier and move more. In the past, you likely beat yourself up because you ate dessert or missed a workout. Instead of thinking you blew it, it's time to realize this was a necessary part of the process that will allow you to find what works.

If you can process these experiences as lessons instead of mistakes, then you will shift your mindset, build your grit, and establish a mental outlook that will help you eat better, enjoy more, and stress less. This means not just removing blame, but also resisting the instant gratification promises made by so many diets. It's the same bait, and it's time for you to accept that the promises of 4-week rapid weight loss are nothing more than an illusion.

Would you rather choose the diet that promises you ten pounds in four weeks or twenty pounds in twelve months? Everyone chooses the shorter timeline, and it's a trap. (And that's assuming the plan can actually deliver on the suggested weight loss.)

In a weird way, the manipulative promises are some of the most accurate aspects of the diets you want to avoid. They are sticking to the short-term because they know it's more appealing to you and because—usually—the benefits start to reverse once all the initial weight loss runs out.

It's frustrating, but if you know that these short-term promises are a trap, you can save yourself many long-term headaches. Remember, every time you go on a bad diet, it does more harm and can increase how much weight you end up gaining back. So stay the course, tap into your grit, and your body will take care of the rest.

CHAPTER SUMMARY

- Embrace an "80 percent good, 80 percent of the time" mentality to reduce stress, enjoy treats, and stay on track.
- Avoid zero percent weeks. The only "mistake" in dieting is quitting completely on healthy habits.
- Changing your perception of healthy and unhealthy foods can help you feel fuller after every meal.
- Your past experiences are the secret to building grit, if you see them as part of the learning process and not that your body is broken. If you reframe your past, then you are in the perfect position to become healthier than ever.

Chapter 7

THE TRAP DOORS

MARION NESTLE IS THE queen of nutrition science. A professor of nutrition, food studies, and public health for more than fifty years, she has won countless awards and long been at the forefront of the science that's trying to make us healthier.

In an interview for *Newsweek,* Nestle—not one to sensationalize—made a big claim:

> *We have now the accumulated evidence, particularly in the last five years, that people who eat more ultra-processed foods have a higher risk of obesity, diabetes, cardiovascular diseases, depression, cancer, renal, and liver diseases. The studies have been overwhelming. There've been hundreds and hundreds of them. There's no doubt that this is not a good thing. It is a problem.*

The term "ultra-processed" refers to the way food manufacturing has changed. And, if you believe Nestle (and many other prominent scientists), it's one of the biggest reasons people have become heavier and unhealthier during the past fifty years.

Ultra-processed foods are the options that now line the interior aisles of most grocery stores. These are the packaged goods that are created with convenience and low cost in mind, which means they are bought frequently and in high quantities.

That's not to say all packaged foods are bad. To understand, it helps to have a basic understanding of the four levels of food processing.

Level 1: Minimally processed

If food comes in a natural form (fruit, vegetables, or animal protein), it's considered minimally processed. It might include minor processing such as freezing or vacuum sealing, which are methods to help preserve shelf life.

Level 2: Processed ingredients

Do you like olive oil? Me too. The consensus is that it's very healthy for you. But it also happens to be a processed food. This level of processing consists of creating a food option from natural food. Whether it's canned coconut milk (from coconut meat) or sugar (from sugar cane), these are forms of processing, but it doesn't mean the ingredient is problematic.

Level 3: Processed foods

Bread, cheese, and canned fish. All can be part of a healthy diet—and all are processed foods. If a few ingredients are combined together, the food is processed. There is more work involved to create these foods, but nothing is added to manipulate how your brain reacts to the foods, which is where problems really begin. Which leads us to level 4 . . .

Level 4: Ultra-processed foods

This is the "if you're eating these foods all the time, then it's time to worry" zone. No food needs to be completely removed, but if there was ever a type of food that causes more harm than good, this is the one. These foods have many ingredients that you know—but they are manipulated to make them taste a certain way that turns you into an eating machine. They are designed to add sugar, fat, and salt in an unnatural way that increases your cravings and makes you more likely to overeat and purchase more. Examples include sugary drinks, cookies, chips, frozen dinners, and some lunch meats.

Eat More, Lose More (The Science of Energy Density)

THE 4 LEVELS OF FOOD PROCESSING

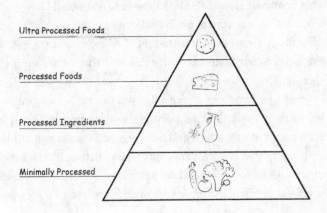

If you eat ultra-processed foods a few times per week, it's not an issue. As much as some dietitians find it cringe-worthy, I openly share my love of Frosted Flakes. I eat them several times a week and love every bite. There's nothing nutritious about it, but I enjoy it and keep it to one bowl a few nights per week. It doesn't disrupt the overall quality of my diet. But one bowl is not the same as several bowls, or days where most of what you eat are ultra-processed foods.

In you believe data on food consumption, we are now eating far too many processed foods spread throughout every meal each day. In fact, research suggests that the American food environment has flipped from one that would help control your hunger (levels 1 through 3 on the food processing chat) to one that is mostly made up of level 4 ultra-processed foods. Studies appear to show that nearly 60 percent of all food purchased is ultra-processed.[1] When that happens, things change from an enjoyable treat that is part of a healthy balanced diet, to something truly disturbing and problematic: eating too many ultra-processed foods are disrupting your brain and gut and making it harder than ever for you to be healthier.

THIS IS YOUR BRAIN ON ULTRA-PROCESSED

Pulitzer Prize–winning journalist Michael Moss is on the hit list of "big food." In his book *Salt Sugar Fat*, Moss shows in great detail "how the food giants hooked us." At the core of his investigative masterpiece is the science of bliss-point foods. These are the ultra-processed foods that are chemically engineered to alter your brain chemistry in a way that would short-circuit your hunger signals.

If you've ever wondered why it seems like you can eat . . . and eat . . . and eat . . . and never get full, the bliss point is the likely reason. This refers to the perfect amount of salt, sugar, and fat designed to make you fall in love with food in a way that is both dangerous and addictive. Instead of eating and feeling full, these foods are a Molotov cocktail of hormonal disruption. The more you eat of them, the more your brain is rewired to want more and more.

Moss's book was defining, but it wasn't entirely damning because research hadn't been able to "prove" the damage of bliss-point foods. That was until a skeptical researcher decided to test a crazy theory.

For decades, research focused on the relationship between calories and weight gain. And time after time, it was clear that the more you ate, the more weight you gained. The missing piece was understanding why some people seemed to eat uncontrollably while others consumed less. And, why did everyone seem to be eating more during the last fifty years?

One theory was the increase in ultra-processed foods. Dr. Kevin Hall—a prominent researcher you met earlier in this book—was skeptical that ultra-processed foods could be the cause. He was on the record calling it "ridiculous" to assume that ultra-processing was the problem. To test the theory, Hall set up a fairly simple study to see what happened when people ate more ultra-processed foods. He had twenty people move into a lab for a month and monitored everything.

One group followed a diet of minimally processed foods, focusing on things like pasta, beef, seafood, and yogurt. The other group ate more processed foods, such as Honey Nut Cheerios, Chef Boyardee pasta, and other packaged foods.

Despite the different food choices, Hall and his team of scientists made sure that each meal had the exact same macronutrient composition. The Chef Boyardee meal would have the same amount of carbs, fats, and protein as the less-processed pasta. The yogurt would have the same amount of protein, carbs, fats, and calories as the cereal and milk. The catch? Participants were instructed to eat as little—or as much—as they wanted, and they were given sixty minutes to eat their meals, three times per day. The study was less about calories, and more about how different types of foods affect how you eat.

At the end of one month, those who lived off the ultra-processed foods gained an average of one pound per week and ate more than 500 calories more per day than those who had the less-processed foods.

Even crazier? Hall and his colleagues decided to see what happened when the participants swapped groups. When those who ate the ultra-processed diet then switched to less processed foods were put on a diet without the ultra-processed foods, they dropped the pounds they gained.[2] In the time that has followed, more studies have backed up Hall's research, which suggests the proportion of ultra-processed foods you eat as a part of your daily meals directly impacts how much you eat. Maybe it should come as no surprise.

In an interview with *Newsweek*, Moss shared that the problem isn't really sugar in dessert-like foods. Instead, it's how the food industry has turned normal foods—like bread and yogurt—into hyper-palatable foods that make you want to eat more and creates an expectation for sweetness in seemingly everything.

So, instead of dessert just being dessert—something you enjoy occasionally— we're being programmed to desire foods that are being transformed into dessert-like treats, and then craving those foods more often. If that wasn't challenging enough, Hall hypothesized that ultra-processed foods cause three primary issues:

1. They mess with your brain chemistry to make you want more food.
2. They are so calorie-dense that you eat significantly more than you think you do.
3. They make you eat your meals faster.

Ultra-processed foods are a problem. But thinking you need to remove all of them and cook every single meal from scratch is not the solution unless you can maintain and sustain it—that feels like deprivation and is unsustainable. As you'll learn in the chapters ahead, if you can use food to outsmart the issues above outlined by Hall, then you can follow a healthy plan without falling into the trap of complete restriction.

WHAT TOOK SO LONG?

You might be wondering why it took so long for scientists to figure out the role of ultra-processed foods. The truth? They really didn't even have a way of measuring the level of processing.

For the longest time, foods were analyzed based on their calorie or macronutrient content (proteins, carbs, and fats).

Then, in 2009, Carlos Monteiro, a researcher at the University of São Paulo in Brazil, created a new way of looking at foods. Called the NOVA Food Classification System, it factored in the level of processing. Ultra-processed foods were those that were modified or made entirely from substances that you could extract from a meal (such as fat, sugar, salt, or starch). The common culprits were the foods you now imagine to be troublesome, such as sugar-loaded sodas, baked goods, salty snacks, and frozen dinners.

Once that happened, it gave a new way for researchers to classify and test foods, and the new findings helped us better understand why overeating seems almost too easy.

WHAT ABOUT GENETICS?

Let's get something out of the way: genetics matter. I want to discuss it because whether or not I say anything, you're probably thinking about it as you consider the type of results you can expect. If you have "better" genetics, it can certainly make it easier to be healthier. But, your genetics don't work the way most people think. Whether it's about a faster metabolism or the ability to lose weight without cutting calories, there are a lot of myths.

If you're going to stop living in the past and playing the same old game, it's time to bury some of the old beliefs that are holding you back from upgrading your health.

Many factors influence how you gain weight. Four stand out in particular:

- HEREDITY: genetics and epigenetics
- DEVELOPMENT: how you're raised, your childhood diet
- LIFESTYLE: behaviors such as exercise, sleep, and stress
- DIET: the foods you eat and your food environment

As you can see, many of these factors are outside your control. You can't change your genetics or how you were raised. Both have a say in how easy or hard the process might be, but—here's the good news—they won't prevent you from getting to the finish line.

For decades, it was assumed that weight loss was a game of chance. There were the haves and the have-nots. Either you had a great metabolism and childhood environment or you didn't. And, if you struggled to become healthier, it was easy to wonder if it didn't matter what you did—you were stuck with the body you have.

Science paints a much different picture. Genetics play a bigger difference in gaining weight and less of a role in losing weight.

There are roughly one hundred genetic markers linked to weight gain and obesity. That's the bad news. The good news? Even if you have one of those traits, it doesn't necessarily mean you're destined to be overweight. Researchers found that people with one of these genes have a 20 to 30 percent higher risk of obesity than those who do not. And if you exercise, you can reduce that percentage.

More important, the genes won't prevent you from losing weight. In a study of 9,000 people, possessing the "weight gain gene" had no influence on the ability to cut body fat. According to the author of the study, professor John Mathers, "Carrying the high-risk form of the gene makes you more likely to be a bit heavier, but it shouldn't prevent you from losing weight."[3]

So there's no need to go back in time or curse the day you were born. Wherever you are right now, you can change your health outcome—which means your best bet is to focus on lifestyle and diet. Notice I didn't say you wanted to reprogram your metabolism. That might be a common reframe, but there's a reason why all your metabolic resets haven't turned you into a calorie-burning machine.

The Metabolism Myths (Yeah, There Are Many)

The first metabolism experiments date back to the early 1600s, when Santorio Santorio (what an amazing name) weighed himself after a variety of acts such as eating, sleeping, working, and even sex. (Who says scientists don't have fun?)

During the past four hundred years, human metabolism has been examined from every angle imaginable, and we continue to learn more about how we burn calories and power our body. But one idea continues to be an almost mythical part of science: the fast metabolism. The idea that you can do something to make yourself burn more calories is so compelling that people have been selling supplements for the last one hundred years with the same promise.

The crazy part? Almost none of it is based on science. You've been taught that a "fast" metabolism is the key to weight loss. You've also been told that your metabolism slows down as you age. You might think your metabolism "stops working" in your twenties, and others will say it's their thirties, or that it was their forties or fifties that finally did them in.

As someone on the other side of forty, I can empathize with the perception. But research suggests much of what we've thought was true was very incorrect. We tend to gain weight over the years. And yes, certain foods just seem to stick to your belly more easily in your forties than in your twenties. But the issue isn't that your metabolism breaks. In fact, it doesn't start fighting against you until you're much older.

A groundbreaking study that combined the work of more than eighty scientists and used 6,500 participants (aged eight days to ninety-five years old) shook the foundations of weight loss. It found that your metabolism is fairly stable from the time you're twenty until you're sixty years old. After age sixty, your metabolism starts to decrease about 1 percent per year.[4] In other words, until you hit your sixties, your body is not conspiring against you for weight gain.

And that's not even the craziest revelation. Raise your hand if you know that heavier people have faster metabolisms.

Yep, it's true. In general, the more you weigh, the more you burn. It all has to do with the energy it takes to run your body every day. We like to think of our metabolism as an on-off switch. You turn it on when you exercise or eat, and it turns off when you're on the couch. In reality, your metabolism is always burning because your body depends on its work. You require energy to think, breathe, and keep your heart pumping. This is known as your basal metabolic rate (BMR), and it accounts for approximately 60 to 80 percent of your metabolism.

As much as it's not ideal to think of your body as a machine (because it turns food into fuel, which is why people stress good versus bad foods), it's a good analogy for your metabolism. Because the bulk of your metabolism is spent powering every movement and action, the bigger the body, the more energy it takes to function.

Some people run "hotter" than others and burn more calories and that helps them stay at a certain weight. But they burn more calories compared to a different person at the same weight. The more weight you gain, the more your body has to work to function. Compare the lean 150-pound person to a 200-pound person and the 200-pound person is going to burn more calories each day from their BMR.

Your metabolism shifts up or down when you gain or lose weight. But extreme diets can break predictable adjustments and recalibrate your metabolism in a way that fights against your goals and makes it easier to regain weight. If you lose weight too quickly, you might disrupt your BMR permanently, which means your metabolism can shut down in ways you can't imagine.

Satan Has a Six-Pack

Trying to achieve rapid weight loss might be a deal with the devil. It's part of the fine print most diets tend to ignore.

When you lose weight, your metabolism slows down. This is not a bad thing—as long as you lose weight the right way. Research suggests that crash diets, such as extreme calorie restriction (like a detox or any plan that cuts too many calories too soon) could have the biggest negative impact on your resting metabolism. In other words, if you lose too much too fast, you might love what you see on the scale, initially. To be clear, both slow and fast weight loss can work for long-term results. But, with rapid weight loss the long-term sacrifice is that your BMR—the bulk of your metabolism—might permanently slow down and make it harder to keep weight off in the long run.

The process is something scientists call "metabolic adaptation." When you lose weight, your metabolism should downshift to adjust for your smaller energy needs. So, if you go from 170 pounds to 160 pounds, it makes sense for your metabolism to adjust too.

Your metabolism can also slow at a much faster rate than the amount of weight you lost. Imagine if you lost ten pounds but your metabolism slowed down as if you lost fifty pounds? Eventually, it would become harder to stay at the new weight. The bigger issue is what happens when your metabolism doesn't recalibrate. Imagine gaining back your weight, and—even though you were heavier—your metabolism wouldn't burn more calories.

This isn't a hypothetical; it's an example of what happens when you give in to extremes. Researchers examined members of the TV show *The Biggest Loser* to understand what happens when you quickly lose a lot of weight. The study, which was published in the journal *Obesity,* examined contestants at the beginning of the show, at the end, and again six years later.

All the participants lost dozens of pounds (one contestant even lost more than 200 pounds). Unfortunately, at the follow-up, thirteen of the fourteen contestants regained a significant amount of weight, and four of them were even heavier than before they started. The most interesting part was the metabolic shift that had occurred. Remember, in a healthy metabolism, the number of calories you burn fluctuates based on your size. The more weight you gain, the more calories you will burn. The more you lose, the more it slows down.

The *Loser* participants, all of whom lost weight quickly, were burning approximately 500 calories less per day than you would expect at their weight. Even though they gained back the weight, their metabolism never reset, which made it harder to lose and easier to gain. Unfortunately, that's only half the story. The contestants also had hormonal changes that would explain why they regained weight.

At the end of the show, the hormone that regulates hunger (leptin) was almost completely depleted. That means their brains were not receiving the chemical that signals fullness when eating, which would leave them in a constant state of hunger. If you think you get "hangry," imagine eating and eating and eating and never feeling full or satisfied? Given the combination of a slower metabolism and low leptin, it's no surprise they gained back the weight. But, it gets worse.

At the six-year mark, after regaining all that weight, their leptin levels were only about 60 percent of where they started before their weight loss.[5] It's not all bad news, but rather a cautionary tale. With weight loss, there is a thing as too much too soon.

On the other hand, there are many other studies suggesting that these types of changes don't happen with all weight loss. The catch is you must be willing to lose at a more gradual pace, which allows your metabolism to adjust with you and help you maintain your new weight.

Upgrading Your Metabolism

Although your BMR makes up the majority of your daily calorie burn, there's still another 20 to 40 percent you can control. The additional calories you burn from your metabolism come from the foods you eat and the exercise you perform.

Your diet influences your metabolism by about 10 to 30 percent, and then exercise—everything from walking to strenuous exercise—makes up the remainder. If you want to burn more calories from your diet, it's important to know that all calories are not created equal. Protein, carbs, and fat are all metabolized differently. Eating 100 calories of protein is different than eating 100 calories of carbs because protein has a higher thermic effect of food (TEF). This is a measurement of how foods are metabolized.

When you eat protein, up to 30 percent of the calories can be burned in the process. In the example above, if you ate 100 calories of protein, roughly 70 calories would hit your body because 30 calories would be burned as a result of the protein's high TEF. Comparatively, carbs have a TEF of just 5 to 10 percent, and fat is usually around 3 to 5 percent. This is one reason higher-protein diets tend to be associated with weight loss and maintenance, and why it'll be a key tool that makes your life easier (and more satisfying).

You might be wondering about "easier" ways to boost your metabolism. After all, there is no shortage of products that promise to boost your metabolism. And it's not just supplements. "Natural" ingredients like coffee, chili, and other spices have a reputation for ramping up your caloric burn. And, on paper, these ingredients technically boost your metabolism, but it's not the type of impact you'll ever see on the scale. Just as adding more gas to a full gas tank won't make you drive farther, making minor changes to your metabolism isn't going to help you burn calories at a rate that makes a difference.

The best metabolism booster is muscle. The more muscle you have—and the less fat you carry—the higher your metabolic rate. The reason is that muscle requires more energy. Remember, the key to a metabolism that works for you (rather than against you) is your BMR. It helps power everything in your body that you're not thinking about, like your heart, lungs, and brain.

It also is fueling the cells in your body. Fat doesn't require much energy. It just sits there and collects dust. It's low maintenance, which is a bad thing and a reason that it's easy to accumulate more of it. Muscle, on the other hand, is high maintenance. It requires a lot more energy when it's at rest, and—when you use that muscle (such as during exercise)—it helps burn more calories too.

To be clear, this isn't about becoming bulky. This has nothing to do with how much muscle you add and everything to do with how much muscle is on your body at any size compared to the amount of fat. Remember the example of the 150-pound person? Genetics aside, if you're 20 percent body fat and 150 pounds, your metabolism is going to burn fewer calories than the person who is 15 percent body fat and 150 pounds. Muscle simply makes you more efficient and helps you process food more effectively.

Diet and exercise are two variables you can control, and soon you'll see how. Now that you understand the common errors that send you down the wrong path, it's time to share a refreshing new way to eat, enjoy, and pick the type of diet that will finally work for you.

CHAPTER SUMMARY

- Limit ultra-processed foods. The more you eat, the more calories you'll consume. A few times per week is okay. A few times per day is not.
- Genetics matters, but they do not prevent you from losing weight.
- Your metabolism slows as you lose weight. This is normal. But, if you lose weight too fast, your metabolism can slow unnaturally. The best "metabolism boost" might be gradually losing weight (instead of rapidly) so your calorie-burn stays higher.

PART 3

YOU CAN'T SCREW UP THIS EATING PLAN

Chapter 8

I WILL TEACH YOU TO EAT

UP UNTIL THIS POINT, everything has been built toward giving you a better path to healthy eating that improves your health and supports your goals, whether that's losing weight, building muscle, or just having more energy every day. We've focused on your mindset, self-perception, common mistakes, trap doors, and even a better diet philosophy. But, you still need to know what to eat and how to make sense of all the endless food options.

As you start to play a different game, you need to reframe your objectives. As we've discussed throughout the book, lots of styles of eating work. It doesn't matter if you prefer lower carbs, intermittent fasting, or counting macros. All of them can work. What doesn't work is following something that you know will be short-lived. Rather than stressing good foods and bad foods—or stressing at all—it's time to embrace food and create boundaries that provide more freedom. Here are your four objectives for healthier eating:

OBJECTIVE #1: Stop trying to be perfect.
OBJECTIVE #2: Eat more satisfying foods.
OBJECTIVE #3: Eat fewer hunger-increasing foods.
OBJECTIVE #4: Include foods you love.

Remember: *You can't screw this up as long as you don't overreact to any meal or food.* To make it easy to accomplish these objectives, here are five simple tools you can apply to your life, regardless of your dietary preferences or restrictions.

SIMPLE TOOLS > RESTRICTIVE RULES

You'll expand your comfort zone by using tools that help you do a better job of eating in a way that keeps you full and provides plenty of variety. That means you can apply the rules to any diet, dietary preference, or situation. Do you prefer to eat vegan? No problem. More of a Paleo-style eater? That works too. Need takeout? Don't stress it.

The five tools outlined below are designed to work with your lifestyle, not the other way around. That way, it'll be easier to build great habits that last. You can truly eat anything every now and then, if you have boundaries and understand how to make the tools work for you.

Don't expect yourself to use all the tools all the time. If you incorporate all of them, you'll have everything you need to accomplish your goals as quickly as possible. Even if you can use just one tool when you're first starting, you're still making progress and doing what's needed to be healthier.

These tools are designed to be the ultimate mind-body combination. Too many plans try to separate physiology and psychology. But, the plans that break you mentally will ultimately fail you physically.

As you work on applying these tools, remember, the goal isn't to have weeks when you're 100 percent—it's to avoid zero percent weeks. Ready to start building a healthier diet? Here are the tools you need.

TOOL #1: Create meal boundaries.

TOOL #2: Prioritize protein and fiber.

TOOL #3: Add a plus-one.

TOOL #4: Take twenty minutes.

TOOL #5: Make takeout (and processed foods) work for you.

Tool #1: Create Meal Boundaries

Today's working world is a model for how our eating schedules are broken. Throughout the last several decades, the workday has become longer. Gone are the days of the 9 to 5. Whether you're in a service position or a desk-worker, overworking is an issue. And this is only amplified by the ways that technology has inserted work into the home. Email and systems like Slack and Microsoft Teams means that we're all always connected, and work is never really over.

The breaking of work boundaries has broken us. Researchers looked at more than two hundred studies during the past twenty years and found that longer work hours are connected to higher incidence of heart problems, poor sleep, health decline, and an increase in smoking, drinking alcohol, and substance abuse.[1] It's not that work is inherently dangerous, it's just that it needs a time and place.

Eating is much the same. If you leave your schedule open to eat at any time, then it's almost too easy to overeat. It's amazing how much over-eating occurs simply because people don't follow set mealtimes. Whether it's snacking on your child's breakfast before you eat or downing a bag of chips while watching late-night TV, a lack of boundaries leads to mindless snacking that can easily disrupt an otherwise good day of eating. That's why creating parameters around when you do and don't eat can be incredibly helpful.

The natural reaction to this suggestion might be, "Wait, are you just suggesting intermittent fasting?" Not exactly.

I used to be a big fan of intermittent fasting. I followed that style of eating for approximately five years, and then I stopped because of two big changes.

1. I became a father.
2. Research showed that intermittent fasting isn't superior to other styles of eating when calories are balanced.

When I became a father, I wanted to be able to enjoy breakfast with my son. I didn't want to stress every morning or fight off food temptation while I would sit with him. I decided the memories of eating with him were more important than any potential benefits of fasting.

Turns out, many of the original benefits of fasting were overstated. The claims of autophagy and weight loss simply haven't stood up when tested—and this is coming from someone who was a huge fasting advocate. If you're eating the same amount in a day (both calories and the types of foods), it doesn't matter if you restrict it to a small window of time or a bigger window. In other words, if having long periods where you don't eat works for you, then do it! But there's no need to feel forced to fast because the amount you eat in a day—whether in 8 hours or 16 hours—maters more than the amount of time you spend eating.

That said, intermittent fasting's greatest contribution might be the structure it provides. Intermittent fasting creates guardrails that make it much easier to follow a plan. Much like having set work hours allows you to clock in and clock out for work, having boundaries for your meals creates a physiological and psychological advantage. The first tool applies to setting an eating schedule based on when you wake up and go to sleep.

How to Control Calories Without Counting Calories

By creating an "eating window," it helps limit the type of unintentional overeating that is common for so many people. The hardest aspect of eating is that it doesn't just occur when you're hungry. You eat with you're bored, stressed, in social situations, happy, sad, and distracted.

From a psychological standpoint, this is where boundaries can help. In the same way that setting a time when your workday is over (don't answer those late-night emails), having times when you eat (and times when you don't) can help provide more control over your day.

Research suggests that simply modifying a start and end time for eating—without doing anything else—can lead to some amazing results. In a UK study, dieters were told to make one change—delay their first meal by 1.5 hours and move dinner up by 1.5 hours. No other adjustments to what they were eating, how often they were eating, or how much. Those who created the boundaries ended up eating less during the short trial.[2]

In another study published in *Cell Metabolism*, people were allowed to select a ten- to twelve-hour window to eat. Similar to the research above, there were no parameters around what could be consumed, just that there was a clear start and end time to eating, and those beginnings and endings could be any time.

The study ran for sixteen weeks. Those who created parameters around their eating lost more than six pounds and were able to keep it off at a one-year follow-up,[3] which is a big deal considering how many people regain the weight.

Again, there is no magic. When studies provide more strictly controlled conditions—such as taking people who have "eating windows" and controlling how many calories they consume and comparing them to an "open eating" structure, in which they eat the same amount of calories—then the weight loss is similar.

But, the question here isn't about calories. We know they matter and will impact if you gain or lose weight. We're trying to implement simple methods that make it easier for you to not overeat, not stress, and not have too much complication. The time limits simply make it easier to stay on plan, and limit times when hunger is not the primary driver of eating. That's why so many people thrive and see great success.

How can you make it work? A simple execution is a two-hour rule that revolves around wake and sleep times. At the start of your day, push back your first meal by two hours from the moment you get up. At the end of the day, stop eating two hours before you go to sleep.

If you wake up at 6 am, then you won't have your first meal until 8 am. Beverages with little to no calories, such as water, coffee, or tea, are all fine. In fact, I'd recommend drinking 16 to 20 ounces of water first thing in the morning.

At the other end of the day, if you normally go to bed at 10 pm, then your goal is to stop eating for the day by 8 pm.

The two-hour adjustment isn't a hard rule. You want to find what works for you. For example, in the test group of five hundred people, some people needed to shift it to one-hour after waking (because of their schedule) and three hours before sleep. The most valuable aspect is having set boundaries, not an exact time frame. But, two hours seems to work best for realistic morning and night responsibilities, and it can help you control early morning hunger and improve sleep.

In general, wake time and sleep time are good end points. While that one study suggested pushing up dinner time by 1.5 hours, this isn't practical for everyone. My family typically eats at 5:30 pm, and it's simply not possible to eat at 4 pm because my children are still at school (and who eats dinner at

4 pm). Not to mention, anything you're doing to improve your health should work *with* your family structure and not create more stress for you or your family. Just as you shouldn't be obsessing about every meal, you don't want your kids to either. And having mealtimes will help create good habits they can carry throughout their life.

Just remember: Don't get caught up majoring in the minor. It's not the specific amount of time you have to eat (no study suggests eight hours is better than twelve hours, for example), and it's not the hour of day when you start or stop (some people think eating at night means your body can't metabolize the food as well and it'll turn to fat, which is also a myth). It's the idea of the boundary and preventing too much late-night eating, which is when a lot of extra calories tend to be consumed.

If you set a "start" and "stop" time for your meals, you will create a structure that puts you in control of your eating, and you will make big progress without adjusting anything else simply because it helps prevent mindless and unnecessary eating and snacking.

WHAT ABOUT AUTOPHAGY?

I wrote a book about intermittent fasting back in 2012 when I was a much bigger believer in many of the claims. One of the biggest alleged benefits is autophagy, or the cellular "cleansing" of your body. This is where your body repairs itself, and there's evidence this can help with natural antiaging and overall health. Fasting is a tool that might support autophagy.

But—and it's a big but—fasting is not the only way (or even the "best" way) to increase autophagy. Much of the research on fasting and autophagy occurs in animal models, such as mice. If you want proven ways to increase autophagy and promote cellular health, your best bets are caloric restriction (eating less), exercise, and better sleep.

There's no research to suggest that autophagy promoted by fasting is better than autophagy from caloric restriction (eating less) or exercise. And, at this point, research would suggest that exercise and eating less is probably more effective. You can fast if you want, but the advantage isn't as great as you might have been led to believe.

SHOULD YOU SKIP BREAKFAST?

Any plan that gives you more flexibility to design what works for you is more likely to succeed. That said, there's more research that suggests skipping a morning meal entirely could be a mistake.

As you saw above, pushing your breakfast back a couple of hours can work because of the guardrails. However, studies suggest that waiting too long might change the way your body processes food. In particular, if you wait until the afternoon and evening to eat, it might negatively impact your metabolism, hunger, and how much energy you burn.[4]

If it works for you to go all morning without food, then that's fine and there's no need to adjust. But there's no need, and it might be advantageous to have some protein in the morning, which leads to the next tool.

Tool #2: Prioritize Protein and Fiber

What if I told you that you could eat three times as much food but not gain any additional weight? It sounds like another gimmick, but this one is actually real. The "secret" is a concept known as energy density, and it's one of the best ways to help you eat more, stay full, and not overeat.

Remember the study about people who ate ultra-processed foods and consumed about 500 extra calories per day? The big takeaway is that when you let people eat as much as they want, they tend to eat more when they are consuming ultra-processed foods. But there's more than meets the eye.

When you look at those 500 extra calories per day, an interesting trend stands out. Almost all the additional calories came from carbs and fat and very little from protein. It seems like some people can eat a lot of food and not gain any weight and not be hungry all the time, while others eat a fraction of the food, gain weight, and are still hungry.

It's not an illusion. It's the real-life magic of energy density. Energy density is a way of describing small amounts of food that are shockingly high in calories. When you eat foods with high energy density, you take in a lot of calories without much food. Low energy density is more desirable for managing hunger and feeling fuller for longer; it's foods that allow you to eat much more without taking in as many calories. To understand, look at the Energy Density illustration.

These two meals have a similar amount of calories, but the meal on the right has three times as much food. The images display how some people can eat more and lose more. The image on the left has high energy density, while the image on the right has low energy density. Learning to appreciate energy density is an easy way to allow you to eat more food while consuming less.

ENERGY DENSITY

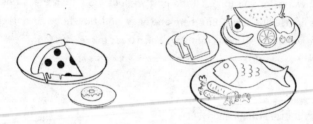

High Energy Density   Low Energy Density

Eat More, Crave Less

Energy density is important because something tricky happens when you lose weight. *As the scale goes down, your brain makes you crave more food.* If you've ever been on a diet and feel like your body is working against you, well, it kind of is. This doesn't happen forever, but it does go on long enough that the cravings make you eat more food and gain back weight.

If you want to outsmart your brain, you need to eat more of the foods that keep you full and prevent your brain from turning into an eating machine. Low energy-dense foods are the key, and the king and queen of those foods are protein and fiber. Studies show a simple but powerful relationship to controlling hunger, managing cravings, and maintaining positive changes to your weight.

The more you increase energy density (eating highly caloric food), the more calories you eat. On the other hand, the more you decrease energy density (eating more protein and fiber, for example), the easier it is to eat less.[5]

Imagine having three different plates of food. All three plates weigh the exact same. The only difference is one plate has the least amount of fat (low energy density), the next plate has twice as much fat—and therefore more energy density—as the first (but weighs the same), and the third plate has three times as much fat as the first (and once again weighs the same). If it were just about the quantity of the food, then you would think people would eat the same amount. But, that's not the case.

This exact concept was tested, and the researchers found that the more fat you added to the plate, the more people would eat.[6] That's not to say that fat is bad—it's a necessary part of your diet. But adding fat is the quickest way to increase energy density, which contributes to eating more. You have more room to eat protein and fiber, but you'll want to be more conscious of how much fat you consume.

Some foods—specifically protein and fiber—will keep you feeling full and satisfied. On the other hand, other options—like carbs and fats—will make you want to eat more carbs and fat.

The (Low Energy Density) All-Stars

If you're looking for foods with lower energy density, here are some of your best options:

- Vegetables
- Fruits
- Whole grains and oats
- Beans and legumes
- Lean meat (such as top or bottom round, sirloin, fillet, or game meats such as venison or elk)
- Chicken
- Low-fat dairy
- Egg whites

The Science of Satisfaction

Despite all the debate about whether carbs or fat make you gain weight (in reality, eating too much of either can be a problem), the real secret is satisfaction.

If you want to satisfy your hunger, start with protein. Not only does it play a key role in keeping you fuller for longer, it's also important to your longevity and healthy aging; plus, the mere act of eating protein helps you burn more calories.

If you recall from the last chapter, about 10 to 30 percent of your metabolism is determined by the foods you eat (known as the thermic effect of food, or TEF). And protein has the highest TEF, ranging from 20 to 30 percent. The more protein you eat, the more calories you burn while metabolizing those foods.

Even better, the more protein you eat, the fewer total calories you tend to consume. One study looked at what happens when you go from a low-protein to a moderate-protein diet. When people doubled their protein intake (from 15 to 30 percent of their diet) they lost 11 pounds . . . without making any other changes. Simply eating more protein increased fullness so people naturally ate almost 450 fewer calories per day.[7] You can hopefully see how all these little changes lead to big results. Eating less ultra-processed foods can save you 500 calories per day. Consuming more protein removes another 450 calories. Those two changes alone could hypothetically save you thousands of calories per week.

The "comfort zone" approach would be to start with protein-packed foods you enjoy. Maybe that's chicken or turkey. It doesn't have to be boneless, skinless, or bland. Just make sure you include it and try not to deep fry it. Maybe you prefer ground beef (burger night, anyone?). If possible, go for at least 90 percent lean. If red meat isn't your preference, eggs are a high-quality protein source. So is dairy, whether that means drinking milk or eating some Greek yogurt or cottage cheese. If you're looking for vegetarian options, dig in on lentils, beans, quinoa, and hard cheeses.

The other part of the hunger equation is fiber. On the surface, it's easy to overlook. Many people typically associate fiber with old age and foul-tasting powders. In reality, fiber stands at the perfect intersection of healthy and enjoyable. It's found in many popular carb-loaded foods, and it easily qualifies as a superfood because of its gut-boosting properties.

The best part? Fiber is a sneaky convenient comfort zone option. Eventually, you'll want to expand your comfort zone by eating more vegetables, not only because they are incredibly good for your overall health, but also because they are a tremendous source of fiber. Even if you don't love vegetables, you can still pack in fiber with some popular food choices. Great places to start are whole wheat bread or wraps (look for options with more than 4 grams of fiber per serving), whole grain pasta, a baked potato, apples and bananas, avocados (1 cup has about 10 grams), nuts (like almonds), beans, and lentils. If those don't sound great, you can also snack on a couple cups of air-popped popcorn or some dark chocolate—both of which have fiber.

Remember the earlier images showing high energy-dense foods compared to low energy-dense foods? It's not that fat or carbs are inherently fattening. It's damaging when either is found in very calorie-dense foods, like the ultra-processed options you want to limit. If you're given those calorie-dense foods, you eat and eat . . . and can't stop eating. It's why people consume an average of 500 calories more per day when eating bliss-point foods.

Wouldn't it be amazing if there were an off switch when you start eating too much? Turns out, there is an off switch, and it's called fiber. When you add fiber to those same foods, it changes the energy density and you eat less food. Fiber wins where a lot of foods lose. Fibrous foods tend to take longer to chew, which helps your brain determine fullness. At the same time, fiber also slows digestion, which keeps you feeling satisfied for longer, so you don't need more food. Fiber also quiets your "hungry brain," which helps shut down cravings.

Fiber might also be the ultimate longevity hack. One meta-analysis of eight different studies found that for every 10 grams of fiber you add to your diet, there was a 10 percent drop in risk from any cause of death. Not bad, right? And if that wasn't enough, researchers reviewed 185 different studies and found that fiber consumption is associated with longevity and other health benefits.[8] Also, when you combine fiber and protein you unlock satisfaction, and that is a strong foundation for any diet that works.

Satisfaction is a concept that's lost in diet culture. Not only do you need to fuel your body, but you also need to be satisfied by eating food you enjoy and then knowing when to stop. That way, your brain can work with you rather than against you to help keep you fuller—and still leave room for you to enjoy other foods, such as protein and carbs.

That's because no single macronutrient is bad or fattening. Rather, you want to limit meals that are too high in both carbs and fats, eat enough protein and fiber to help prevent your brain from lapsing into food zombie mode. (If you want to make someone gain weight, just reduce how much protein and fiber they eat.)

That's the common thread in research. You don't need to eat a super-high amount of protein. But, when protein levels drop too low, hunger tends to increase and weight seems to follow. Starting in the 1960s through the early 2000s—a period when the average American became larger and larger—protein consumption decreased while carb and fat content increased.[9]

This Is Your Brain on Ultra-Processed Foods

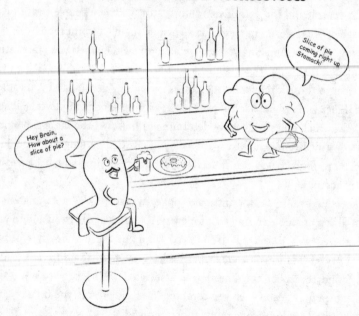

If you believe it's a coincidence, science paints a picture of what might be happening. Your body may have an unlimited ability to consume and store carbs and fats. This is seen in studies that focus on over-feeding. When people overeat, the extra calories rarely come from protein. Instead, it's typically from eating more fats or carbs.

Unfortunately, we are designed to store a lot of fat. Blame evolution if you want, but the capacity for fat storage is almost unlimited. And this is why hunger is complicated. Because your capacity to store energy is unlimited, the ability to overeat is almost too easy—unless you know how to control your hunger.

Cut Me Off, Bartender

Although your body is fueled by calories, your hunger is controlled by satisfaction.

Hunger is all about communication between your stomach and your brain. It's a bartender–patron type of relationship. Your stomach is at the bar ordering drinks. Your brain is the bartender.

When you eat foods that are designed to stimulate satisfaction and fullness, your body sends a signal to your brain telling you to cut yourself off. No more food for you.

When you eat foods that aren't designed to satisfy your hunger—which is different from satisfying your taste buds—the bartender will keep on serving. This is how we become food drunk, eat too much, and wonder why no one stopped giving you food when it was clearly time to cut you off.

If you do a good job of including protein and fiber—they should fill up, at least, 50 percent of your plate when having a meal—then there are plenty of ways to eat other foods you enjoy and not overeat.

WHY AM I NEVER FULL?

Does it seem like you always have room for dessert? The way you build your plate might make it more likely to eat more when you should be full.

A variety of flavors can trick your mind into thinking you can eat more, even when you'd normally be full. It's called sensory-specific satiety. "Fullness" can be sensory-specific. In other words, you might not want to eat any more food of a specific flavor (sweet, salty, or so on). But when you introduce a new sensory experience, your body "magically" finds more room for it.

For example, if you have a mix of sweet and savory foods, you'll be able to eat more of both, but focusing on one type of flavor helps you hit your fullness level sooner. While there are certainly savory and sweet desserts, most of the good stuff will have a combination of sweet, savory, and salty. Once you turn to dessert, you're likely to eat more of it, regardless of what you had for your meal. So, the real magic is what happens before dessert.

In one study, people ate a four-course meal. *Those who ate the same type of food for all four courses consumed almost 60 percent less food than those who ate different foods.*[10] This can even work with foods you enjoy. Vox Media tried to re-create this research by having people eat a lot of mac and cheese. Once they were full, participants were then offered either more mac and cheese or ice cream. When offered more cheesy goodness, their interest dropped from a six (on a ten-point scale) down to a one. Even though participants had the same level of fullness, once offered ice cream (instead of mac and cheese), they ate *three times* as much food. The point? You really do have a second stomach for dessert. So, if you just "eat until you're full" at dessert, you're likely to overeat.

How do you avoid this? For one, you can use science to your advantage. When eating vegetables, research suggests that having a variety of vegetables helps children eat more of them[11] (if it works for kids, it can work for you too!). Combining carrots with greens will help you eat more of both. Next, lean on the protein and fiber. They'll help you feel satisfied and full. The next part is trying to ensure you maximize the flavor of your meal without having too much flavor variety.

As you'll see in Tool #5, not every night will be dessert night. So the real key is filling up and not automatically assuming you need dessert. (Because, remember, even if you're full, your "dessert stomach" will be able to handle more.) But when you want dessert, try to add a little natural sweetness to the meal to help curb your hunger when you move to dessert. This can be as simple as adding a serving of sweet potatoes, adding fruit into a salad, or drizzling a little honey into a marinade. This helps reduce how much you'll eat for dessert, because research suggests that we desire a food more when it introduces a new flavor.

By simply understanding how fullness works, you can make sure your decisions and freedom to enjoy work with you—and not against you. That way, you can enjoy your dinner—and have your cake too—without fear of turning into a bottomless pit.

Tool #3: Add a Plus-One

Do you prefer carbs or fats? It's not a trick question because there is room for either—or both—in any diet.

After you select protein and fiber, the next step in building a healthy plate is thinking about your food preferences. It might seem different to think you even have a say in what you eat when we're talking about dietary plans, but—remember—this game is built around compliance, sustainability, and some enjoyment. If protein and fiber are the parts that expand your comfort zone by presenting you with something new and unfamiliar, then the carbs and fats you choose should be within your comfort zone.

The idea of the "plus-one" (more on this in a moment) comes down to a fun question: Do you want more bread and pasta (carbs) in your life, or are you more of a cheese and peanut butter (fats) fan?

I recommend eating meals that consist of three steps:

- Step 1: 1 to 2 servings of protein (the size of the palm of your hand)
- Step 2: 1 to 2 servings of fiber (fibrous carbs, the size of the palm of your hand)
- Step 3: 1 to 2 servings of a "plus-one"

A "plus-one" is the addition of either carbs or fats. Every meal is an opportunity for you to enjoy either one. The catch? It's in your best interest not to eat a lot of *both* carbs and fats in any given meal.

When you serve high amounts of carbs and fats together, it becomes easier for you to overeat. For one, as mentioned, you can store both carbs and fats in almost unlimited quantities. And, when you combine them in high amounts, you also create energy-dense meals. This means eating less overall food while consuming more calories, which you want to avoid. The plus-one is the key to keeping variety that is so often lost when trying to eat well.

You'll learn about the serving sizes soon, but you might be wondering, "How do I decide if I should have one or two servings?" I want to emphasize that the goal is to eat as much as possible of the satisfying (low energy density) foods, and then adjust to help you see the changes you desire. There are two factors to consider: the number of meals you eat per day and your goals.

If you eat three or fewer meals per day, then you'll want to focus on two servings per meal of protein and fiber, and then adjust your plus-one amount based on your hunger. If you're eating four or more meals per day, then—because you're eating more often—you might be better suited sticking to one serving.

Keeping the number of meals you eat in mind, then you'll adjust quantities based on your goals. If you're trying to lose weight, I recommend keeping your protein levels higher. That means, sticking with the two servings of protein per meal. With protein set, follow the guidelines for meal frequency that I just shared (two servings of fiber and plus-one if you eat three meals or less).

If you're not seeing changes after one or two weeks (remember, be patient!), then reduce your plus-one down to one serving per meal. This should lead to changes. If you stall, again—be patient!—and see what happens. As we'll discuss more, plateaus are a part of the process. You won't lose weight every week. But, if you're stuck, reduce your fiber down to one serving in the meals where you are *least* hungry. You still want to prioritize fiber and maximize satisfaction, so make small changes rather than big ones. You'll be surprised how the slight adjustments can lead to surprising results.

The opposite is true if you want to gain weight and build muscle. Focus on enjoying two servings per meal of each of the categories. And, if your weight isn't changing, you can always add in another meal, or bump up to three servings of protein and fiber in your meals.

DON'T MAJOR IN THE MINOR

Sometimes, when you add a plus-one carb source, there will be a little bit of fat. That's okay. Fat is not bad.

And, sometimes, when you add a plus-one fat source, there will be some carbs. That's also okay. I will provide more guidelines to help simplify the process, but—in general—know that you don't have to sweat every ounce of food that goes into your body.

Putting It All Together

As a general rule of thumb, I prefer to avoid counting calories because I'm terrible at math . . . and because the minute eating becomes about numbers, it can easily become stressful or create anxiety. That's not to say you can't count calories; it certainly works. But you don't need to count calories, track foods, or stress exact macros to be successful.

That said, numbers are an inevitable part of eating. You can't go grocery shopping without seeing labels that highlight calories, sugar, protein, fat, and carbs. And, in a world of packaged goods, it helps to make sense of what you see. Otherwise, you might stare at a label and still feel stressed, which is the opposite of what we want. So, I'm going to walk you through the numbers behind the plan.

The numbers are not the goal. *You don't need to count a single calorie.* You can use your hand to measure anything. But, if you struggle recognizing foods for what they are (whether they are a carb/fiber, fat, or protein), this will make your life easier.

If you're looking at labels, build your foundation by selecting foods within the following ranges:

Step 1: Protein

PROTEIN FOUNDATION = 15 to 40 grams minimum (you can have more protein, but 15 grams is a good lower limit)

Step 2: Fiber

FIBER FOUNDATION = at least 4 grams of fiber within about 15 to 30 grams of carbs

Example: You might eat two slices of bread that total 30 grams of carbs and 5 grams of fiber. This is not a plus-one carb source. This is still just part of your foundation.

Step 3: The Plus-One

This is when you can add more carbs or some fat. Again, if you need ranges, here's how you can picture creating a meal that works for you.

ADDING FATS: If you're adding a portion of food that has more than 5 grams of fat (ideally 5 to 15 grams of fat), then consider it a plus-one fat source. Keep in mind, this is the amount of added fat. You might have some fat from the foundation of protein and carbs or some from using a little cooking oil, and that's okay.

ADDING CARBS: If you're eating more than 15 grams of carbs (within a 15- to 35-gram range), then that's a plus-one carb source. Adding something with 10 grams of carbs? Don't overthink it. You're talking about 40 calories. You can't stress every little thing you eat and expect to be successful.

Making the System Work for You

Enjoying a burger is a perfect example of how to make the plus-one system work for you. If you want to eat a burger and fries, then you'll want to cut back on fat on your burger (because the fries will be your plus-one carb). If you want a juicier burger (think adding bacon or cheese or guac), then you'll want to hold off on the fries (because the additions to your burger are a plus-one fat).

Here's how it might work:

Hamburger Plus-One Carb Version
Protein: Hamburger (ideally >90 percent lean meat)
Fiber: Whole wheat bun
Fat: From the burger
Plus-One Carb: Two handfuls of French fries

Hamburger Plus-One Fat Version
Protein: Hamburger (ideally >90 percent lean meat)
Fiber: Whole wheat bun
Fat: From the burger
Plus-One Fat: Added cheese

The Finer Details

Because people love examples, I'll outline below how very different meals can all work on this plan. The sample meals are just ranges. There is room to roam outside of them, but they give you an idea of how it works and show that *every meal doesn't have to be the same.* Some meals can have more food, others a little less. Each variation, while different, allows you to eat comfortably. Remember, the "foundation" is just the combination of protein and fiber.

Types of Meals

Foundation + Higher Carb + Lower Fat
- Protein: 20 to 60 grams
- Carbs: 40 to 60 grams (at least 4 grams of fiber)
- Fat: 5 grams

Foundation + Lower Carb + Higher Fat
- Protein: 20 to 60 grams
- Carbs: 20 grams (at least 4 grams of fiber)
- Fat: 20 grams

Foundation + Moderate Carbs + Moderate Fat
- Protein: 20 to 60 grams
- Carbs: 30 to 40 grams (at least 4 grams of fiber)
- Fat: 10 to 15 grams

Example Meals

Chicken Breast + Pasta Marinara
Protein: Boneless, skinless chicken breast
Fiber: ½ cup of whole wheat pasta
Fat: Olive oil in the marinara sauce
Plus-One Carb: Additional ½ cup of pasta (for a total of 1 cup of pasta)
Sirloin Steak (cooked in butter) + Baked Potato
Protein: Steak
Fiber: From baked potato
Fat: From sirloin steak
Plus-One Fat: Added butter to steak and potato

Fish Tacos
Protein: Fillet of fish
Carbs: 1 whole wheat tortilla + veggies

Fat: ¼ avocado
Plus-One Carb: 2 handfuls tortilla chips

Rice Bowl with Chicken, White Rice, and Veggies
Protein: Boneless, skinless chicken breast
Fiber: ½ cup white rice + veggies
Fat: Cooked in ¼ tablespoon of olive oil
Plus-One Carb: ½ avocado

Scrambled Eggs, Bacon, and Toast
Protein: Eggs
Fiber: 2 slices of whole wheat toast
Fat: From the eggs
Plus-One Fat: 2 slices of bacon

Why Dieting Is Like Dating

Meet Sarah. She lives in Manhattan, works six days per week, and loves carbs. She was told by her favorite Instagram influencer to limit carbs, so she's been trying different low-carb diets. In general, she can maintain a low-carb life for about four to six weeks. She loses weight and feels great, and then things go sideways. Next thing she knows, she's camped out at Lilia, an amazing Italian spot in Brooklyn. She consumes more than she normally would, sees the scale shift the next morning, and then thinks carbs are the problem. Next thing you know, she's eating far too much at every meal because she *thinks* she has to be strict all the time. What she doesn't realize is that when she completely restricts something like carbs, scale fluctuations are normal and not reflective of "real" weight gain.

Sarah's problem isn't carbs. Or Lilia. If she ate, drank, and slept normally after her amazing meal, the scale would've returned to where it was and potentially gone lower with time. The issue is the belief that she can't eat her beloved carbs in the first place. Instead, it's helpful to think of healthy eating like dating. You wouldn't choose to be in a relationship with someone you despise from day one, so why would you do that with the foods you eat?

You can build a healthy diet that's higher-carb or lower-carb. "Do what works for your body" is simple advice, but it works incredibly well. You have a different body from your friends and siblings, so why wouldn't you want to make personalized adjustments that fit you best?

Anything that sounds like it would make your life miserable is going to be a problem. Because while your body might survive just fine, your mind won't. You will quit the plan, you will learn to hate nutrition, and you'll probably end up more confused and a few pounds heavier than when you started.

This is why a plus-one is so powerful. Change is hard, but it's made easier by familiarity and enjoyment. This is how you expand from the yellow part of your comfort zone into the green.

WHAT ABOUT EXTRA PROTEIN?

If you want to eat more protein, that's fine. Every food has limits, but protein is the hardest macronutrient to convert into fat. For vegans, there aren't that many straight sources of lean protein that don't also have carbs or fats. This is not a problem, but it also means that adding more protein usually means adding a plus-one carb or fat.

Tool #4: Take Twenty Minutes

In the book *Switch: How to Change Things When Change is Hard*, authors Chip and Dan Heath argue that businesses struggle to get the most out of their employees because they lack clarity. They argue that for employees to be confident and motivated, they need to know exactly what changes to make—and see them make a difference—in order to keep doing them.

The same thinking applies to how you eat and why so many restrictive plans become popular. But not enough plans make it clear what keeps you feeling full and satisfied. People see that extreme plans appear to make a difference, so they're willing to go through misery. But as we've discussed, those methods are designed to stop working, create a bad relationship with food, and make it harder for you to lose weight after you stop the plan.

If you want to be confident that what you're doing is working, one of the changes you can make immediately—without going shopping or changing your food preferences—is the amount of time it takes for you to eat a meal. This is one of the most effective habits of people who have a good relationship with food, lose weight, and maintain weight loss.

When you eat too fast, your body doesn't have enough time to process the food and realize if you've had enough. I told this to the five hundred people who tried this plan, and most of them almost laughed off the idea of this making a difference. But once they tried it, they realized how quickly they were eating their food and how *taking more time immediately helped them eat less*. So before you skip to the next tool, I encourage you to let this one sink in because it's one of those behaviors that can change everything.

Your body needs about twenty minutes to process hunger. We've talked about how hunger is very much a brain-driven process. Your brain depends on signals from your body, and that includes everything from the chewing process to the amount of time it takes for your stomach to signal that you're full.

Research suggests that eating slowly increases food satisfaction, boosts fullness, and promotes the gut hormones that help with satiety.[12] And that's only half of the equation. It's not just how much time you take to eat, but also your level of awareness about what you're eating.

Studies show that distracted eating—if you're on your phone or watching TV—also increases the amount of food you consume in a meal.[13] It's a perfect storm of a lack of attention, poor memory, and changing brain signals. Your hunger responds not just to the food in your belly but also to visual cues. When you're distracted, your brain doesn't get these signals, which increases the likelihood that you'll want more food.

Eating slowly gives your system time to work the way it's intended, so your body can send signals letting your brain know when you've had enough. Taking more time also leads to fewer issues with your gut health and helps prevent overeating.

How much can twenty minutes save you? At least 70 calories per meal, more than 200 calories per day, or more than 1400 calories per week.

That was the takeaway from research from the University of Rhode Island. Their study focused on slow versus fast eating. In the study, women were instructed to either eat as quickly as possible or to put their utensils down between bites and take more time chewing.

The fast eaters finished eating in nine minutes. The slow eaters took twenty-nine minutes. While you might assume an extra twenty minutes of eating would result in significantly more calories, the slow eaters ate 70 fewer calories. There were no other differences, and the scientists even made sure that both groups drank the same amount of water (because hydration can affect fullness).[14]

Slowing down is a small change that makes a big difference. But you don't even realize how quickly you eat until you set a timer and force yourself to take at least twenty minutes to enjoy your food.

How to Eat Slowly

Consider yourself warned: This will be harder than you think, because you likely eat much faster than you've ever realized.

If you're looking for a simple technique to help keep yourself accountable, you might want to borrow a tactic that comes from General Stanley McChrystal, a retired four-star general who once led the United States Joint Special Operations Command, which oversees units like the Navy SEALs and Army Rangers.

According to author Eric Barker, McChrystal gets his soldiers to execute at the highest level by following the simplest of steps. He communicates the following:

1. Here's what I'm asking you to do.
2. Here's why it's important.
3. Here's why I know you can do it.
4. Think about what you've done before.
5. Now go and do it.

Eating isn't anything like war, but it might be time for you to have a similar conversation with your body. Imagine it going like this:

1. I'm asking you to take twenty minutes to eat each meal.
2. You need to make it a priority because until you remove your distractions you'll keep struggling with hunger, your health, and your weight.

3. I know you can do it because you set aside twenty minutes for things that are much less important, like social media and TV.
4. You have done things that are much harder than slowing down during meals. This isn't hard; it just requires commitment.
5. Don't make the same old mistakes. Set a timer—and commit to the small things that can make a big difference with your health.

Tool #5: Make Takeout (and Processed Foods) Work for You

Did you know that fewer than 40 percent of Americans say they enjoy eating? It's a troublesome number, especially when you consider that as a society we're eating more than ever.

Enjoyment has dropped significantly since the late 1980s, according to Pew Research.[15] And that lack of enjoyment is strongly tied to several different factors, including our love of cooking (or lack thereof), eating out, and exercise.

While the same number of people still cook meals at home, they're doing it less often. And that means the number of people who now eat at restaurants has dramatically increased. The same Pew data suggests that 33 percent of people eat takeout at least once per week and another 33 percent eat out at least twice per week.

So why is the enjoyment gone? When you dig deeper, the reason might be because you're too stressed about what you're eating, spending too much time feeling guilty about your meals, and perceiving you're eating the wrong types of foods, especially when having takeout. It's time to bring back enjoyment by changing your relationship with the food environment.

More Freedom, Less Guilt

How do you eat healthier when the foods you desire are "forbidden," and the foods you're "forced" to eat only make you want to eat more of the forbidden foods?

The answer: Make the "forbidden foods" part of the plan so they are no longer forbidden.

It'd be great if you could cook every meal. And if you do, that's wonderful. I recommend that you try to cook as many meals as possible, and the recipes in this book are designed to be quicker, easier, and enjoyable. However, it's not realistic for most people. We live in a culture where takeout is a part of our food environment, ultra-processed foods are everywhere, and it's unlikely that you can live your life without ever relying on the convince of processed foods.

If you want what you can't have, then allowing yourself to have takeout food—with certain boundaries—can help you make better choices and eat less. In general, you can safely eat out two or three times per week (if you follow the takeout guidelines in Chapter 9), without much concern. You can eat out more than that if needed (remember I figured out that I was struggling with my weight during my years of travel because I was eating takeout five times per week), but the more often you eat out, the harder it can be to avoid the temptation of the more calorie-loaded options.

The previous tools still apply to takeout and ultra-processed foods. But, unlike many other plans, there will be room for you to eat these foods without the guilt.

Make Processed Foods Work for You

It's helpful to remember that not all processed foods are created equal. What really matters is limiting the ultra-processed. These are the foods that seem to send you on a detour to the land of endless eating.

Ultra-processed foods are a problem—and the poison is in the dose. You don't need to go full restriction. In fact, if you could shift that to even 20 percent of your diet, the results would be dramatic. It's a domino effect of hunger.

The less often you eat ultra-processed foods, the less you crave calorie-dense foods, thereby making it easier to shut off your hunger. That result is less overeating and more time in your comfort zone.

To recap, most ultra-processed foods manipulate sugar, fat, and salt. These three ingredients create a "bliss point" that causes your brain to go wild for the types of food you want to limit or avoid. In general:

- Bliss-point foods are loaded with calories and are high energy density.
- Those calories act like brain control and turn you into a bottomless pit of hunger. Your body has more than 10,000 tastebuds. And when you

eat bliss-point foods, you trigger all of them to the point that your body says, "I'll have seconds . . . thirds . . . fourths . . . and fifths."
- Ultra-processed foods also make you eat faster, which is part of the reason it's easy to overeat.

The goal is to be more in control so that you can intuitively follow your hunger and cravings and give your body what it wants and needs. To help accomplish that, it is good to have boundaries that help you control eating.

To be on the safe side, it's best to limit your ultra-processed intake to *once per week*. This doesn't mean you can only have takeout once per week (more on this in a moment). Instead, it's giving yourself space to enjoy ultra-processed foods. This includes things like:

- pop/soda and fruit drinks
- sweet or savory packaged snacks (think cookies or chips)
- candies and cake mixes
- butter substitutes (margarine and spreads)
- energy drinks
- pre-prepared pies, pasta, and pizza dishes

SIMPLE CALORIE CONTROL

Eating healthy isn't always easy, but some tips can be simple. Here are two that help.

1. MINIMIZE LOW-PROTEIN LIQUID CALORIES: Everything from fruit juices and sugary sodas to wine and spirits. This isn't to say that you can never drink these; you just want to limit how often you have them. Non-caloric drinks, such as coffee, tea, and naturally sweetened beverages (think flavored waters) are fine.

2. MINIMIZE SNACKING: Some of the healthiest countries in the world never snack. If food reward is part of the reason we overeat, limiting the number of times you eat can make meeting your dietary goals much easier. Plus, most snacks tend to be low in protein and fiber, which makes it harder to feel full. And, despite what was popular in the early 2000s, eating more often does not boost your metabolism, so you're not holding yourself back.

YOU'VE GOT THIS

It's natural to look at the list of ultra-processed foods and wonder if you can pull this off. But there are many reasons why this doesn't have to be as hard as you think.

You Have Many Takeout Options

As you're about to see, you also get to enjoy restaurants. When you're not restricting as many foods, your psychological cravings aren't as intense. So maybe you're not eating baked goods, but there are other foods you love that will fit into the plan and leave you satisfied without feeling restricted.

Your Diet Tools Will Change How You Feel

Every tool that you just received will help manage your physiological cravings. You're used to being hungry because of how you used to eat. But when you start combining protein and fiber and taking twenty minutes to eat, you'll experience a massive difference. How you have typically felt on a diet is not how you will feel this time though. When you're more satisfied, cravings and food temptation dramatically change.

Life Is Easier When You Treat Yourself

You're shifting from "never eat this food" to "have it once or twice per week." This subtle shift takes the edge off eating, removes pressure when you indulge, and allows you to enjoy treats more because there's no guilt associated with every last calorie. Not to mention, when we think of dessert, it's easy to believe that ultra-processed foods are all that exists. But there are plenty of other desserts you can enjoy. Within this book, you'll find a dozen different options that you can make, and even some packaged goodies you can still eat.

Your Food Preferences Will Change

Your body's reaction to ultra-processed foods changes when you eat less of them. This is why the comfort zone approach is so important. It's hard to go cold turkey. It's easier when you gradually reduce certain foods.

When you start eating fewer ultra-processed foods, you reduce your cravings for them. That's because those foods are engineered to override your brain's ability to signal when you're full. Your current expectation of eating is based on your current temptation to eat these foods. The less you eat of them, the more your brain works to support you (not work against you). When that happens, you'll feel more in control.

The 200-Calorie Lesson

Sugar is not the same as cocaine, despite what some people will try to convince you on social media. But understanding why people think they operate the same way can help you create an environment in which you don't eat like an addict.

You have a pleasure center in your brain (it's called the nucleus accumbens, if you're curious) where things like dopamine make your brain light up and want more of whatever makes you feel good. Cocaine triggers the release of dopamine. So do sugar and many other bliss-point foods. But you know what else releases dopamine? Listening to music you love, going outside, getting a raise, and—as you might expect—sex.

In fact, research shows that all food triggers a dopamine response.[16] It's why food is so enjoyable. However, cocaine—unlike other pleasure triggers like food or sex—binds to your dopamine receptors and breaks the normal cycle of how your brain functions, so the dopamine stays in your system longer, meaning you want more and more to maintain that same prolonged high. This does not happen with food, which is what makes cocaine very different.

Few areas study dopamine more than addiction, so to make you less of a dopamine monster, it's helpful to pull a page from the addiction playbook. And that means controlling your environment.

"One of the best things you can do to help your diet is to control your cues," says Stephan Guyenet, Ph.D., author of *The Hungry Brain*. Guyenet explains that temptation is a much bigger problem than hunger.

"Your reward path is very simple. If you walk past a pizza store, smell cookies in a kitchen, or see the food you love on the counter, all of them can trigger the release of dopamine, push you towards the behavior you want to avoid, and cause you to eat foods you're trying to limit," says Guyenet.

Controlling hunger doesn't have to feel like mission impossible. You have the tools to do it. But environmental triggers can override the system and make you eat more, even when you're highly motivated to stick to a plan. That's why it's essential to control your home environment as much as possible.

Researcher Pierre Chandon found that if you want people to eat healthier, it's not about how you describe food or whether you put it on a smaller plate. It's whether you make that food more or less accessible. By his estimates, moving certain foods farther away can easily save you more than 200 calories per day.[17]

This has been replicated in workplace research. In one study at Google, snacks were placed either close or far from a beverage station. When the snacks were close, men ate twice as many snacks and women's snacking went up by one-third.[18]

The two hundred–calorie lesson isn't about the number of calories you save—it's about remembering your environment controls how much you eat. If you want to have more comfort, create a more comfortable environment. As Guyenet explains, it's not just moving them farther away. It's limiting accessibility and making it harder for you to get them.

If you know there's ice cream in the fridge, you're probably going to eat it. Sure, it's not in sight, but it's not hard to get to it, either.

The goal isn't to control everything. It's to turn your home into a place of limited temptations. That means doing your best to limit the number of ultra-processed foods to a few items. This could mean cookies or other baked goods being in your home but stored in a place that's not easily accessible.

I have kids. They eat treats. But the ultra-processed foods are kept out of their reach—and ours. That way, they get to enjoy them when they've been earned, and my wife and I can't simply eat them every time we walk by the pantry.

If you're going to keep food out or have it accessible, focus on foods that are filling and less tempting. This means options like fruits, vegetables, seeds, and nuts. If you walk by an apple and don't eat it, it's probably because you're not hungry.

If you walk by a box of cookies, you might not be hungry, but you know how you'll feel after eating it. That's the dopamine trigger that helps you "find" your appetite, eat the cookies even though you didn't want them, and wonder how it happened.

WHY TAKEOUT IS BETTER THAN DINE-IN

Eating takeout is the perfect comfort zone exercise. On one hand, you need to challenge yourself by eating at restaurants less often and making smarter choices (you'll see options for the fifty most visited restaurants in Chapter 10). And you also get to live in your "comfort zone" because having convenient options are not forbidden, which means as you build new behaviors you're not doing so with extreme, restrictive behaviors that lead to stress. And if limiting stress and temptation is a key to better eating habits, then you might want to limit how often you dine at restaurants. That's because going to restaurants increases the likelihood that your willpower will fall apart with each passing entree.

When you order takeout—rather than eat at restaurants—you remove cues that can make you overeat and avoid many excess calories, whether it's the extra bread or chips that are served before you even order.

Again, there's nothing wrong with bread or chips on their own. You might not even want them, though, and the sight and smell easily make you order them, eat them, and then eat some more. It can be a gateway into eating much more than you want.

HOW TO PERSONALIZE YOUR PLAN

There's a reason this book is called *You Can't Screw This Up*. It's because there isn't one correct way of eating, you have lots of flexibility, and mistakes aren't really mistakes. A good diet requires a level of personalization that makes you comfortable because that allows you to be consistent, eat well in a sustainable way, and see the benefits. And, as you see benefits, your behaviors will strengthen and evolve as long as what got you to your destination in the first place doesn't break your will.

Part of the problem with many diets is the fixed style of eating. It's difficult to change someone's food preferences overnight because one person's dream meal might be something another person dreads.

The five tools you've been given are a way to navigate the foods you eat. They provide a structure for what should be on your plate (you'll get plenty of examples in the next chapter), suggestions for how to feel full, strategies to use if you're craving more carbs or fat, tips that work with your brain (instead of against it) to control hunger, and enough flexibility to help you navigate the food environment when you don't have time or energy to cook.

Still, there are so many little details and preferences to consider that it's worth taking the time to pause and walk through different scenarios, questions, and concerns you might have.

What About Food Allergies and Dietary Preferences?

If you have a food allergy or sensitivity, you should feel comfortable adapting to your food preferences, whether that means avoiding animal proteins with a vegan or vegetarian diet or cutting out gluten (if you have celiac disease) or dairy (if you are lactose intolerant).

Whatever you've heard, none of these foods are bad. For most of us that don't have an allergy or disease, they are a choice. Gluten doesn't make you fat. Neither does dairy. But if you don't like the way you feel when you eat those types of foods or you have other reasons to avoid them, then remove them from your diet.

Can I Eat the Same Thing Every Day?

Read enough social media conversations and you'll undoubtedly hear this claim: "I ate eggs every day and they made me fat," or, "I used to drink a whey protein shake after every workout, but now I have food allergies and can't drink any protein." You glance at your scrambled eggs and wonder, "Can I give myself food allergies?"

Rest assured, if you eat the same thing repeatedly you won't build up resistance to it. The American College of Allergy, Asthma, and Immunology states there is "no relationship" to eating foods repetitively and developing an allergy.[19]

Can I Drink Alcohol?

Many studies have shown light to moderate amounts of alcohol—such as one or two drinks, a couple times per week—do not necessarily lead to weight gain.[20] From a weight gain perspective, alcohol is processed in unique ways. Your body has a harder time storing alcohol and the 7 calories per gram it delivers[21] (more per gram than carbs and protein, but less than fat). So, instead, your body fast-tracks that booze through your system.

Additionally, a high percentage of calories from alcohol get burned up by your metabolism. The thermic effect of alcohol is about 22.5 percent, which is more significant than carbs and fat. All of which is to say a little bit of alcohol won't necessarily make or break your weight loss goals, so you can enjoy the occasional wine, drinks with friends, or beers while watching your favorite sport.

This doesn't mean alcohol is good for you or will support your health goals; it's not and it won't.

For starters, heavier drinking (more than two drinks in one day) is associated with weight gain[22] and increased waist circumference,[23] as well as poor health. Excessive alcohol consumption is the third-leading cause of premature death in the United States.[24]

Some research suggests the problem isn't necessarily the alcohol itself but what can come along with drinking, whether it's the 83 grams of sugar hiding in your frozen margarita or the insatiable hunger that follows. A review published in *Physiology & Behavior* found that, sure enough, drinking before or during a meal tends to increase food intake.[25]

What's your move? If you want to enjoy the occasional glass of wine or cocktail, treat it like your plus-one. As long as you're still eating protein and fiber, using the other tools, and not drinking every night, you should be able to strike a healthy balance. My recommendation is to limit your drinking to once or twice per week (at most), and control the number of drinks you enjoy.

CHAPTER SUMMARY

- You don't need to be perfect with the five tools. Use them to help you know when to eat (your boundaries), what to eat (prioritize protein and fiber), how to eat (slow down and take twenty minutes), and why there's no need to overthink what you enjoy (whether that's carbs, fat, takeout, or the occasional treat).
- Build meals around protein and fiber. They will maximize satisfaction and reduce cravings and hunger.
- Allow yourself ultra-processed foods once per week. If it happens more than that, don't sweat it and overreact or feel guilty. Keep using the tools. One bad meal or a bad week will not break your health.
- Your food preferences matter, and that's why the plus-one exists. You can follow any style of eating you prefer. Just use the five tools to help guide your behaviors and embrace your food preferences, allergies, or limitations.

Chapter 9

LET'S ORDER TAKEOUT

IF YOU'VE EVER WATCHED *The Simpsons*, you've probably witnessed an episode where the lovable Homer Simpson tries to negotiate with his brain.

Homer's conscious works overtime trying to prevent him from saying something compromising. In one episode, Homer's wife, Marge, asks him: "What did you do last night?"

Homer to his brain: "Don't say drink beer, don't say drink beer, don't say drink beer."

Homer to Marge: "I drank beer . . . DOH!"

We laugh because Homer just can't seem to help himself, but you might be wondering what this has to do with eating takeout. In words that Homer would appreciate: If you want to outsmart the doughnut, you have to stop telling yourself to avoid doughnuts.

Restaurants make it harder to eat healthier. And whether you know a lot about nutrition or couldn't identify a protein from a carb, it's difficult for everyone. But we need to stop telling people to never eat at restaurants, because it's like Homer negotiating with his brain.

As I admitted at the beginning of this book, just because you know how to make healthy choices doesn't mean it's easy when you're ordering at a restaurant. In fact, the lack of guidance around how to enjoy takeout makes it harder for everyone. The USDA conducted a massive review on the impact of "food away from home." (It's the fancy name for takeout.)

Among their findings:

- People with the most nutrition education don't order healthier options (even when you control for dietary awareness and food preferences).
- When you eat more calorie-loaded foods away from home, you don't compensate by making healthier choices later.
- In fact, when you eat takeout, the typical trend is to eat even more food over the course of the day. In other words, the number of total calories you eat in your non-takeout meals increases on the days you have takeout. (This is possibly due to the impact of the bliss-point foods on your hunger.)
- Dieters have more trouble ordering takeout, struggle to order healthy food, and because they are restricting, are more likely to splurge on calorie-dense foods.

Add it all up, and the researchers calculated that just one takeout meal per week leads to an average of gaining roughly two extra pounds per year.[1] It doesn't have to be this way.

RETHINKING TAKEOUT

Years ago, my wife was asked if she would rather give up food or sex for the rest of her life.

She chose sex. (This wasn't when we were arguing about the paint on the window, although that probably would've made me feel a little better about her response.)

As much as it stung, my wife isn't alone. When I surveyed one hundred people and asked them the same question (partially to calm my own insecurities), 82 percent said they would also give up sex and choose food. We are social creatures, and food is much more than what you eat to survive. It's culture, friendship, celebration, mourning . . . and can even be a love language.

Learning to add takeout isn't about eating whatever you want. It's about enjoying the conveniences of modern food, and not feeling like every takeout meal is a dietary sin. Every day of your life you have menus. There are foods you can buy at the store. If you fill your cart with only cookies, you know the outcome. But, if you fill your cart with lots of good options and throw in a box or two of cookies, there's no reason you can't be perfectly healthy.

Your job is to learn to navigate the takeout menu the same way. There are a few common ways restaurants add loads of unnecessary calories to their foods. If you can limit those, then you've won half the battle. It's the freedom you want to eat many of your favorite meals.

If there's a holy grail of nutrition, it's finding ways to make delicious foods convenient, less energy-dense (more protein and fiber, less fat), and affordable.

On the surface, this is no easy task. A study in *JAMA Internal Medicine* found that the average meal from independent restaurants and small-scale chains contain more than 1,300 calories.[2] That's far too many calories. But, when you take a deeper look, many of the issues with the calorie-loaded items on restaurant menus are linked to the unnecessary addition of fats and carbohydrates.

Remember, fats alone are not a problem. Neither are carbohydrates. It's a combination of high-fat and high-carb (especially when mixed with low protein and fiber). And, when you review many of the most popular dishes at restaurants, it's not the primary ingredients that are the problem. It's the addition of extra fats from cooking oils, and extra sugars and carbs from sauces and marinades.

You don't need to completely remove the oils and marinades. But turning down the amplitude on the fat and carb bath not only saves you hundreds of calories, but also fundamentally changes the nature of the meal, which affects how much you eat.

HOW TO ORDER (AND ENJOY) TAKEOUT

"Give a person a fish, and you feed them for a day. Teach someone to fish, and you feed them for a lifetime."—proverb

It's time to grab your hook and reel. To set a ground rule: Eating out effectively isn't a free-for-fall. You'll need guardrails to prevent you from being your own worst enemy. Everything else is straightforward. Apply the two steps below to any meal, and then follow the recommendations when you order takeout.

There's no need to be perfect. If you want to order differently, chalk it up as a bliss-point meal, enjoy, and then continue with the plan. I'll remind you again and again: The only way to screw up is to act like you've screwed up, punish yourself, and stray completely from the tools you've been provided. One meal is one meal. Follow the takeout guidelines most of the time, then those days when you step outside the lines your body won't care. Here's your guide to ordering takeout.

Before You Order

Set Your Plan

The most successful goals are both doable and clear. Start by creating a plan for how often you'll order takeout. A good range is anywhere from one to three times per week. It'll make it easier to decide when to have takeout and when to cook. Home-prepared meals are still the foundation of a good plan—let takeout meals fill the gaps.

Request an Oil Change

Request that your dishes are made with one-fourth (a quarter) of the oil. You can make this request on any takeout app or if you call the restaurant. Added fat from oils is one of the strongest contributions to why we as a society have gained more weight.

You might wonder if they'll actually use a quarter of the oil. Probably not. But, my experience is that the request (just 25 percent of what you normally use) gives the cook or chef a very good idea that you only want a very little amount of oil. I've ordered two identical dishes: I asked for the oil change on one and then compared it to the normally prepared dish. You can see a noticeable difference (less greasy and oily), but the flavor is not lost.

Limit the Sauce

Request all dressings and sauces in a container. Ideally, you'll use half of the single container that's provided. For example, the average Caesar salad dressing container has approximately 4 tablespoons of dressing, which is more than 300 calories. That's like adding a kid's meal to your salad. We want to keep the flavor without being unnecessarily indulgent. You can still eat the entire dish and cut down on excess calories.

HOW TO THRIVE ON TAKEOUT

No matter your restaurant preference, this guide will help you navigate the menu and stay in your comfort zone.

Sushi

A lot of the sushi rolls can be surprisingly high in fat, which is not a problem on its own. But, when you consider that sushi is loaded with rice, that combination of carbs and fats can cause you to overeat. Here are ways to enjoy.

- Sashimi with a side of rice
- Rolls that do not include tempura
- Grilled meats or fish with rice
- Nigiri sushi
- Meat and vegetable dishes cooked in broth

Your Takeout Order

Select one or two cut rolls or nigiri and let the rest of your meal be the sashimi of your choice. You might love tempura, but it's not your best bet unless it's your bliss meal for the week.

Mexican

The name of the game is grilled. Grilled chicken, shrimp, steak salads (but not taco salads with the fried shell). Try a grilled carne asada, chicken, or shrimp plate with salsa, veggies, and rice.

Your Takeout Order

Tacos and fajitas—either three tacos or one order of fajitas. The key is limiting your condiments and not going crazy on things like sour cream, queso dip, and cheese. Get these elements in a small container and use them to add flavor.

Choose black or kidney beans over the refried options. And, as much as it pains me to say it, don't start the meal with chips.

Indian
Lots of Indian dishes rely on amazing spice blends for flavor—including fresh fish dishes, chicken, tandoori, lamb, and beef kabobs and skewers. Avoid sauces and marinades.

Your Takeout Order
Tandoori will be your best friend, and opt for yogurt sides. If you love coconut milk, we're going to recommend holding off on those dishes. Most curries are also a trap door.

Italian
You can enjoy pasta and be healthy too! The secret is how you mix and match your favorite noodle with other proteins. When selecting your meal, salmon and other fresh fish dishes, filet mignon, roast chicken, grilled mussels/clams, grilled prawns, grilled calamari, vegetable side dishes, salads, veal, and chicken piccata or scaloppine are all good choices.

Your Takeout Order
Pick your pasta of choice but stick with marinara or pomodoro options. Limit cream sauces like Alfredo. Frutti di mare will be hard to beat. Looking for an appetizer? Skip the bread and go for minestrone soup.

Thai
Enjoy Thai steak or chicken salad, chicken or steak satay, grilled fish, shrimp, or squid with rice noodles or white rice, fresh spring rolls (wrapped in unfried rice paper).

Your Takeout Order
Think one appetizer plus one main. Rice noodle options such as pad see ew and pad krapow will work well. You can go with pad thai, but specify that

they should use a quarter of the oil. Some restaurants will load it up with 1,000 calories of oil alone. And stick with ordering a single dish—which can be tricky with Asian cuisines.

Chinese

Go for grilled Chinese chicken salad, steamed vegetables, baked/grilled/ steamed fish or prawn dishes, vegetable soups. No sweet-and-sour dishes (definition of high carb plus high fat). No fried dishes.

Your Takeout Order

Go with one appetizer and one main. Choose steamed dumplings or "summer" rolls instead of fried wontons or egg rolls. Summer rolls are made with thin rice paper and usually contain fresh vegetables and shrimp or lean meats like chicken or pork. If you can avoid the fried stuff, keep sauces on the side, and oils at a minimum, Chinese cuisine tends to have a great combo of proteins, veggies, and starchy carbs from rice or noodles.

Brunch

A satisfying brunch can set you up for a fun and active day. Egg dishes are going to be a go-to option, but you don't have to feel limited. You can enjoy things like sausage, bacon, or pancakes, as long as you're not combining all of them together.

Your Takeout Order

Build your perfect breakfast by using Tools 2 and 3. Start with eggs, and then choose your plus-one by either adding meat (think bacon or sausage) OR a side of carbs (whether that's a single pancake, toast, or English muffin).

Mediterranean/Seafood Restaurants

These restaurants can be some of your best options because of how many dishes prioritize lean sources of protein. Go for grilled or broiled fish (salmon, ahi tuna, whitefish, monkfish, and so on), grilled sea scallops or prawns, mussels, salads and vegetable sides, lean meat kabobs/skewers, and a side of rice. You'll want to limit fried options such as calamari.

Your Takeout Order

Select your favorite type of fish or seafood, add a steamed vegetable, and combine it with rice, a baked potato, or some fresh bread.

THE PIZZA RULE

There's a reason you love pizza. It has the perfect (or imperfect) combination of ingredients to create powerful cravings. Simply put, pizza is a bliss-point food. That means it's best to limit it to once per week (and don't assume you can have it three times and consider it a regular takeout meal). But there's no reason to avoid it. Pizza is a personal favorite, so every Friday is pizza night for my family. We order in, enjoy it guilt-free, and try to limit other ultra-processed foods for the week.

Chapter 10

THE ULTIMATE TAKEOUT MENU

Eating at the Top Fifty Restaurants in America

THE FIRST RULE OF takeout is there's no need to feel guilty about takeout.

That is the overriding theme of this book, and it continues in this section. I want you to feel free to make orders that you know reflect the tools you've been given without wondering if something mysterious is lurking in your meals. Restaurants are masters of positioning something that's healthy (like salad) and loading it with thousands of calories.

It'd be great to know if you could comfortably order certain items without worrying that every restaurant experience is a bliss-point meal. The point of this chapter is to show you which options you could eat, on any given day, without worrying about whether it hits your needs for protein, fiber, carbs, and fat.

This chapter includes recommendations from the top-fifty most-visited restaurants in the United States, listed in alphabetical order. When you go through the guide, you'll pick up on certain themes that will, hopefully, help you order more effectively anywhere. These aren't the only foods that fall within the comfort zone, but they're the options that you can confidently order.

No matter what you choose—or even if you step outside the guardrails and make it a bliss-point meal—remember to avoid any guilt, slow down when you eat, enjoy, and then get back on track.

Applebee's

Sirloin (8 oz.) + Grilled Veggies

Hard to beat steak and veggies. It's a classic meal for a reason, and Applebee's doesn't screw this one up. The sirloin is a leaner cut and the veggies add a good mix of fiber and fat, without going overboard.

Thai Shrimp Salad

Another reason to praise shrimp! This entree is another great example of how a popular seafood can work perfectly to create a flavorful dish that's loaded with protein, fiber, and healthy fat.

Cedar Salmon with Maple-Mustard Glaze

Applebee's does a lot of things that inflate the calories of some meals, but they do a good job of not messing up the classics. Just like the sirloin, this salmon dish is exactly what you want: an entree that has added flavors but not at the cost of going crazy with added fat and sugar.

Arby's

Classic Roast Beef

It's rare when a signature meal can be a go-to option, but that's the case with Arby's roast beef. Yes, you're technically tempting the bliss-point gods with the mixture of salt-fat-carbs (it's low in sugar), but if you stick to the sandwich and avoid fries, you're looking at more than 20 grams of protein and less than 400 calories, which is something you can make work for you.

Classic Roast Chicken

Much like the roast beef, this meal pushes the boundaries without crossing them. Yes, it's higher in sodium, which can trigger hunger. But it's also a protein-packed meal that is less than 400 calories. For added flavor, ask for the Buffalo dipping sauce because the added spice can help curb hunger.

Turkey Sliders (x2)

Any time you get something with a slightly smaller portion, it's an opportunity to double up and have a filling meal without going crazy on calories. That's exactly what happens with the turkey sliders.

Bojangles

Bojangles isn't as much of a calorie-bomb as many other restaurants, as the majority of their options cap out around 600 calories (with some exceptions). However, they don't have any options—literally not one—with a good amount of fiber, and there isn't any easy way to add more fiber. The options below are still good, but if you eat at Bojangles, be sure to increase your fiber consumption the rest of the day.

Grilled Chicken Sandwich (no mayo)

About half of the calories (let that sink in) come from the mayo. As I've mentioned, I don't like mayo, so it's easy for me to remove. If you want it, take a small spoonful, spread it on, and enjoy it without a second thought.

Grilled Chicken Salad

It's not exciting but it gets the job done with grilled slices of chicken breast served on a bed of fresh romaine lettuce, iceberg lettuce, and red cabbage, topped with cucumber slices, shredded carrots, grape tomatoes, and monterey cheddar cheese.

Oven-Roasted Chicken Bites

Consider this rotisserie chicken without all the work. These tender nuggets of chicken breast don't look like much, but they're pretty good.

(Note: You're probably wondering about the chicken tenders? If you're going that option, the four-piece homestyle tenders are your best bet.)

Buffalo Wild Wings

Brisket Tacos

A sleeper item on the menu. The brisket tacos are full of flavor, give you everything you want from a BBQ restaurant, but without consuming thousands of calories.

AB Favorite: Naked Tenders + Potato Wedges

The Naked Tenders are almost pure protein. Match with the smoky adobo or medium signature sauce, and then feel free to order the regular size potato wedge to add carbs, fat, and fiber.

Boneless or Traditional Wings (six count) with Dry Seasoning + Carrots and Celery (no ranch)

Don't worry, you can still eat at Buffalo Wild Wings and have wings. Whether you prefer traditional or boneless, the key is sticking with the six count, and then add carrots and celery for the fiber boost.

Burger King

Tendergrill Chicken Garden Salad

Some fast-food salads are loaded with up to 1,500 calories, but this isn't one of them. Not only is it lower in both carbs and fats, but it has a good boost of protein and a few grams of fiber to give your body what it needs to stay full.

Breakfast Burrito Junior

The title might say junior, but this is still an adult-size meal. This breakfast burrito has balanced amounts of protein, fat, and carbohydrates for a satisfying meal.

Whopper Jr.

The Whopper is a fan favorite, but the portion sizes are usually what pushes things overboard. Go the Junior size, slow down, and enjoy.

Carl's Jr.

Charbroiled BBQ Chicken Sandwich

Of all the chicken sandwiches on the list of top fifty restaurants, this one might be the best. It's likely because most chicken sandwiches opt for mayo, whereas the BBQ adds some sugar but significantly less fat and fewer calories, which means you get to enjoy this meal.

The Big Hamburger

Carl's Jr. is known for its burgers, but most of them should be enjoyed infrequently. The exception? The Big Hamburger. It might be basic, but it's still a delicious burger that you don't have to make yourself, and it tastes pretty good.

Chicken or Beef Soft Taco + Guacamole

If a restaurant offers tacos, it's usually a pretty safe option. Both the chicken and steak tacos are low-calorie and high in flavor. Add a side of guac to bump up the fiber and fullness factor and you'll be good to go.

The Cheesecake Factory

When I saw this restaurant on the list of top fifty restaurants in the United States, it felt like it would be the biggest challenge. It's not easy to find options at a place that seems to pride itself on calorie counts that are as big as the menu itself. But they do exist, and you'll be pleasantly surprised with your options. As always, the option exists to just make this a bliss meal. After all, the cheesecake at Cheesecake is very good. (A suggestion: If you're getting a salad, just go with the basic "tossed green salad" on the appetizer menu and add chicken, shrimp, or salmon. Almost every other salad is a 1,000-calorie meal masquerading as a bed of greens.)

AB's Favorite: Grilled Steak Medallions

This meal is so good that I can't believe it's less than 500 calories. But that's what happens when you know how to pair flavors with red meat. It also comes with a side medley of asparagus, shiitake mushrooms, cherry tomatoes, and mashed potatoes. If you like steak and you're at the Cheesecake Factory, this is hard to top.

Seared Tuna Tataki Salad

It's not on every menu, but it should be. When you cut the dressing in half, you're talking about a high-protein, fiber-packed meal that you could eat every day.

SkinnyLicious Chicken *or* Shrimp Soft Tacos

They might have a misleading reputation, but tacos can be a staple of any diet. The mix of protein, fiber, and fat—with endless options and varieties—makes this a great option. Cheesecake does satisfaction right by packing in 12 grams of fiber and more than 30 grams of protein for either the chicken or shrimp option.

Chick-fil-A

Chicken Tortilla Soup

You might not even know Chick-fil-A has soup, but it's really good and incredibly underrated. With more than 20 grams of protein and 17 grams of fiber, it might be the most filling soup you've ever tried.

Bacon, Egg, and Cheese Muffin

It doesn't sound like it would be good for you, but this option is full of surprises. It checks all of the boxes for fat, protein, and carbs, and it's delicious.

Grilled Chicken Sandwich

With less than 7 grams of fat and more than 20 grams of protein, one's hunger will be satisfied at 380 calories.

AB Favorite: Eight-Count Grilled Nuggets + Small Waffle Fry

The grilled nuggets are available in five, eight, and twelve-count. Each works, but the eight-count is your sweet spot because keeping it at eight means you're getting the amount of protein you want—and you can order a small waffle fry. And who doesn't like waffle fries?

Chili's Grill & Bar

AB Favorite: Chicken *or* Shrimp Fajitas

This is my go-to when I'm on the road and need a dish I can trust. There seems to be a Chili's in every major city, and this is about as reliable of a dish as you'll find.

Guiltless Grill: Sirloin (6 or 10 oz.), Grilled Chicken Salad, *or* Mango-Chile Chicken + Glass of Wine

Sometimes, the "healthier" options are nothing more than window dressing. But three of the options at Chili's do a great job of prioritizing protein and fiber, not going crazy on both carbs and fat, and keeping calories in check so you can enjoy a glass of wine.

Chipotle Mexican Grill

Chipotle gives you the option to customize almost anything, so you'll want to design your meal using the tools you've been given. Reference these guidelines the next time you visit.

- Pick a protein—any are fair game.
- Add your fiber: Your two best choices are beans *or* guacamole.
- Add your plus-one. This depends on what you selected in Step 2.

If you choose beans, then you have two options: add carbs with *either* rice or a tortilla (but not both) *or* add fat with *either* cheese, sour cream, or guac (but not multiple options).

If you choose guac, then you need to focus on another carb source rather than fat because the guac—while good—is calorie dense. Add *either* rice, beans, or a tortilla.

- To top it off, add veggies and salsas.

Cracker Barrel

AB Favorite: Good Morning Breakfast

This is the simplest selection on the menu because you don't have to make any additional choices. Load up on protein from the egg whites, fiber from the fruit, and soul food flavor from the grits.

Old Timer's Breakfast with Fried Apples and Turkey Sausage

The hardest part of Cracker Barrel isn't the delicious homestyle cooking. It's that many of the entrees play nice . . . and then the additional sides are where all hell breaks loose. If you want a fulfilling breakfast, order the Old Timer's and pair it with apples and turkey sausage.

Bowl of Chili + Side Biscuit

When in doubt, look for the chili. This bowl packs 12 grams of fiber and more than 25 grams of protein and leaves you room to enjoy one of Cracker Barrel's delicious biscuits (choose this over the cornbread).

Culver's

ButterBurger "The Original" (single) + Broccoli

Give a little, get a little. If you want to dig into Culver's signature burger, it's best that you add a little green into the mix. The Original burger does a good job of blending proteins, carbs, and fats, but it's missing fiber. The broccoli has you covered.

Strawberry Fields Salad with Grilled Chicken

It's true that fast-food salads just don't always taste that good. This one keeps enough flavor by adding fruit while staying under 400 calories. And it's the only salad that checks the box for added fiber.

George's Chili

Another restaurant with a great chili option. It has more fiber than any other dish (that's not also loaded with more than 1,000 calories), with almost the same amount of protein as the burger.

Dairy Queen

Rotisserie-Style Chicken Bites (eight count) + Small Fries

With 100% white meat, the Rotisserie-Style Chicken Bites are a good choice with 34 grams of lean protein. Low in carbs and fat, this meal allows you to order fries to give you added fiber and fullness.

Grilled Chicken BLT Salad

Dairy Queen's Grilled Chicken BLT Salad is moderate in fat, low in carbs, and packed with protein and some fiber. In terms of dressing, opt for the Light Italian.

Grilled Chicken Sandwich

There is only one sandwich on the menu that comes in at fewer than 20 grams of fat, and this is the option. Order up and enjoy!

Del Taco

Carne Asada *or* Grilled Chicken Taco Del Carbon, Guac'd Up, x2

Someone told me this is a new offer. I had admittedly never tried Del Taco before, but I was glad to include it. These are low enough in energy density that you can enjoy two if you please. Mix carne asada or chicken with onions, cilantro, and guac in a corn tortilla.

Del Combo Burrito

Burritos can be difficult because of all the different elements—wrap, protein, beans, cheese, and sauce. Somehow they pulled this one off while staying under 500 calories, which is a job well done.

Denny's

Build Your Own Grand Slam: Hash Browns, Fruit, Egg White, and Bacon

Energy density works, which is why you can still enjoy Denny's "choose your own adventure" version of the Grand Slam. The egg white scramble provides the protein (but saves you fat), the bacon adds extra protein and fat, and the hash browns and fruit give you a dose of carbs and fiber.

Build Your Own Burger: Grilled Chicken on a Brioche Bun with Avocado, Red Onion, and Tomato

I'd never tried a burger at Denny's before, but the combo of the bun with avocado, red onion, and tomato hits the spot.

Wild Alaska Salmon with Dinner Bread and Broccoli

If you didn't know that you can order wild Alaskan salmon at Denny's, you're not alone. But it's a healthy option that checks all the boxes for a very filling meal.

Domino's

As you know from the Pizza Rule (see page 145), the deliciousness of takeout pizza is something that can only be enjoyed so often. Homemade or frozen options tend to be the better way to go. But if you're ordering from Domino's, these are your three best options:

- 3 slices of thin-crust pizza
- 2 slices of regular-crust pizza
- Personal pan pizza

Dunkin'

Chicken, Bacon & Cheese Croissant Stuffer

Sounds decadent, but with less than 400 calories, you're getting a balanced meal of protein, carbs, and fats, all without taking in much sugar.

AB Favorite: Veggie Egg-White Flatbread

An egg-white patty omelet and cheese, with diced red and green bell peppers, mushrooms, and green onions, all on a multigrain thin.

Bacon-Topped Avocado Toast

The bacon says unhealthy. The avocado screams healthy. The reality? Blindly labeling foods is overrated, and this meal gets a thumbs up.

(Note: You're probably wondering, "What about the doughnuts?" They're all delicious, and they're best left as a weekly bliss-point meal.)

El Pollo Loco

AB's Favorite: Double Avocado Salad—Chicken *or* Shrimp

These two items are part of El Pollo Loco's "Fit Menu." I've already discussed how those lists can be deceiving, but these meals were another pleasant surprise. If I was cooking my own meal, I couldn't ask for a better mix of protein, fiber, and fat.

Fire-Grilled Chicken (chicken thigh) with Black Beans

I prefer chicken breasts, but I know many people love the thigh. Too often, though, restaurants will use the thigh (which has more fat) and cook it in so much oil that it becomes a calorie bomb. That's not the case here, so you can enjoy the thighs and mix in some beans for the fullness.

Fire-Grilled Chicken (chicken breast) with Corn

Nothing against the thighs, but this is more my speed. The dish is almost identical to the option above, but you're picking the breast instead of the thigh and opting for corn instead of beans.

Firehouse Subs

Small Cajun Chicken Sub (half the mayo)

It's not quite a grilled chicken sandwich. The Cajun flavoring completely changes the experience from your typically grilled chicken meal. A bulk of the calories are in the mayo, so make sure they go easy.

Engineer (not Fully Involved)

This sandwich has a little bit of everything: smoked turkey breast, melted Swiss, and sautéed mushrooms. They offer it "Fully Involved," which means adding mayo, mustard, lettuce, tomato, and onion. My take: Being a little less involved does more for the sandwich. Drop the mayo and mustard, keep the vegetables, and you'll enjoy the flavor combination of the mushrooms, Swiss, and turkey.

Chopped Hook & Ladder Salad

Yeah, it's a salad at a sub place, but it's too good of an option to leave off the list. The Hook & Ladder is a popular sandwich option, and this salad gives you all of it—smoked turkey breast, Virginia honey ham, romaine, tomato, bell pepper, cucumber, mozzarella, pepperoncini, and dressing—but without the bread.

Five Guys

While Five Guys is a personal favorite, it doesn't have as many takeout-friendly options as other fast-food burger places. For me, it becomes a bliss-point meal because I'd rather enjoy the greasy food that dances around the limitations of the menu. But if you're trying to stick to the plan, there are two options you can make work.

Little Hamburger

The burgers at Five Guys are a good blend of 80/20 meat (the protein/fat ratio). The problem is that the bun runs higher in fat than most other places, and Five Guys is known for stacking two burgers into one bun. The solution? The Little Burger sticks with just one patty and helps keep the calories at a manageable level.

Veggie Sandwich

This is not a veggie burger. As the menu explains, it's "freshly grilled onions, mushrooms and green peppers layered with lettuce and tomatoes on a soft, toasted sesame seed bun." It's a little lower on the protein side, so for the extra boost, go with the cheese variation.

Hardee's

Big Roast Beef

There aren't many sandwiches or burgers here that meet your needs, but the Big Roast Beef is one of the exceptions to the rule.

Bean, Rice, and Cheese Burrito

If you can sneak beans into an item, it tends to be a little more nutrition friendly. And that's exactly the case with this vegetarian option, which supplies more than 20 grams of protein.

Chicken Bowl

I have a strong bias toward bowls, but that's just because they're convenient, blend flavors well, and are easy to adjust to your needs. You can order this with or without the cheese.

IHOP

Build Your Own Omelet
The key to making this entree work: Hold the sausage and cheese and stick to vegetables, bacon, and avocado.

AB Favorite: Two Scrambled Eggs + Choice of Turkey Bacon *or* Ham (two pieces) + Sourdough Toast
It's not officially a "build your own breakfast" option, but the best way to order at IHOP is to call your own shot. These each come as a side, and you can combine them together to create a great, satisfying meal.

Three Buttermilk Pancakes + Ham + Scrambled Egg White
If you want to dig into the signature dish (the pancakes), it just requires a little creativity. Get a short stack of the pancakes (which have a good amount of fiber), and then pair them with ham and egg whites for the protein boost.

In-N-Out Burger

Hamburger with Onion (use ketchup and/or mustard instead of spread)
A lot of people disagree, but I think In-N-Out is one of the most overrated restaurants in America. I don't think the food is bad, I just think it's over-hyped. That said, the Hamburger with Onion gets the job done and even has a few grams of fiber to keep you satisfied.

Cheeseburger with Onion (use ketchup and/or mustard instead of spread)
Just like its sister option, if you love cheese on your burgers, add it to your meal and enjoy!

Jack in the Box

Chicken Fajita Pita (with whole grain pita)
For 320 calories, the Chicken Fajita Pita has more than 20 grams of protein paired with 4 grams of fiber. Getting both veggies and whole grains is a win-win. This is also the lowest in sodium compared to all other chicken

options, which means you reduce the likelihood of hitting the sweet spot of ultra-processing that can make you ravenous.

Grilled Chicken Salad

The Grilled Chicken Salad is a balanced meal that doesn't require you to tear out ingredients like many other sneakily calorie-loaded salads. It's low enough in both fat and carbs that—if you're feeling like it—you could even add a kids' serving of seasoned curly fries.

The Burger

We did a double-take when reviewing the nutrition on the entire menu. But, after checking (and checking again), the lowest calorie entree on the entire menu is the Jack-in-the-Box Burger. At only 270 calories, it's a little lower than you'd ideally want on protein, but there's enough to keep you full.

Jersey Mike's

It's worth mentioning that you can get any sub as a "tub size," which is a fun way of saying "we'll scrap the bun and put all the fixins in a plastic tub." You can do that if you want, but if you're going to a sandwich shop, I figure you want to—ya know—eat some bread.

Natural Turkey Sub Regular Size (no olive oil)

Oil has high energy density and adds a lot of unnecessary calories to meals that already have enough energy. This sub proves it. Remove the oil and save yourself approximately 250 calories; it's a perfectly balanced meal.

AB's Favorite: California Dreaming Regular Size (no olive oil)

Just as with the Natural Turkey Sub, if you cut the olive oil, you completely change this sandwich. The mix of guac makes it delicious and hard to beat. When on the road once, I ate this three straight nights for dinner.

The #4 Regular Size (no olive oil)

You've probably noticed the trend, but once again hold off on the olive oil. The mix of meats and cheeses provides so much flavor and protein that you won't even notice it's missing.

Jimmy John's Sandwiches

At Jimmy John's, you have lots of freedom to turn anything into a lettuce wrap. Assuming you want a sandwich with bread, here are your go-tos.

Slim 2 (roast beef) or Slim 4 (turkey) Eight Inches on French

Jimmy John's offers a variety of "slim" options, but each can differ by hundreds of calories. Your two best bets are the roast beef or the turkey, both of which come in around 400 calories (compared to the others that are around 600 calories).

Big John on French Bread

Anything named "Big John" sounds like it's going to be too much, but this option manipulates its nutrition in a good way by mixing higher fat with moderate carbs and protein.

AB's favorite: Turkey Tom (sub avocado spread for mayo)

This is my go-to option. I swap out the mayo because I think mayo is disgusting (convenient for me from a dietary perspective, and no judgment for those of you who love it), and the avocado saves you calories and fat, and adds additional fiber.

KFC

Kentucky Grilled Chicken Breast with Corn Bread and Side Salad

Kentucky Grilled Chicken Breast is protein-dense with 38 grams, has no carbs, and is low-fat. That means you can set this meal up like a plus-one option. Add the cornbread (it has 11 grams of fiber!), add a side salad, and your body will be satisfied.

Original Recipe Chicken Breast and Corn on the Cob

Who said all fried food has to be off-limits? While many fried options tend to run up the fat content, that's not the case with the original recipe chicken breast. The meal is packed with nearly 40 grams of protein, and by adding corn on the cob, you get your plus-one carb and fiber.

Kentucky Grilled Chicken Drumstick (x2), Green Beans, and Macaroni Salad

Kentucky Grilled Chicken Drumstick is relatively low-calorie, so you can grab two of them and still have room for two sides that will give you fiber, flavor, and vegetables.

Little Caesars

Once again, the pizza rules are in effect.

Longhorn Steakhouse

Flo's Filet (6 oz.) + Steamed Asparagus *or* Steamed Broccoli *or* Two Slices of Wheat Bread

Once again, the filet is going to be a cut of choice when dining at a steakhouse. To make sure you get fiber, opt for the asparagus, which packs 5 grams in your side dish. If you're not an asparagus fan, the bread is another good option.

Renegade Sirloin (8 oz.) + Steamed Asparagus *or* Steamed Broccoli *or* Two Slices of Wheat Bread

The other steak of choice is once again the sirloin cut. You can get a slightly bigger portion than the filet for a similar amount of total calories. Same suggestions apply for the added fiber.

Longhorn Salmon (7 oz.) + Steamed Asparagus *or* Steamed Broccoli *or* Two Slices of Wheat Bread

If you're not feeling like steak, salmon is your next best option. With a similar protein and fat combination (but without the red meat), you'll have a very filling meal and room to select a side.

McDonald's

Snack Wrap (Ranch Snack Wrap, Honey Mustard Snack Wrap, Chipotle BBQ Snack Wrap)

The Snack Wrap is a calorie-controlled balanced meal. Each wrap mixes 20 to 30 grams of carbohydrates, with 9 grams of fat and about 20 grams of protein. Whatever dressing preference, you're coming in below 300 calories with less than 6 grams of sugar.

Premium Southwest Salad with Grilled Chicken

You're probably not heading to McDonald's craving a salad, but if you find yourself there, it's a good option. It's one of the most fiber-loaded options on the menu, which means if you order hungry, you should end up full.

Premium Grilled Chicken Classic Sandwich

Save the crispy version for a bliss-point meal. By choosing the grilled over the crispy, you save 13 grams of fat and turn a hunger-inducing meal into something that's more likely to leave you satisfied.

Olive Garden

Create Your Own Pasta

When you're in control, it's easy to stay in the comfort zone. Here's your best bet:

- Select angel hair or spaghetti
- Add chicken or shrimp
- Ask for half the marinara sauce

AB's Favorite: Shrimp Scampi

Shrimp is a great option at almost any restaurant because it's high in protein and low in every other macronutrient, so it's easy to pair. This dish—whether on the lunch or dinner menu—hits the spot.

Herb-Grilled Salmon + Breadsticks

The Olive Garden might be best known for their breadsticks, but things can get out of control fast when pairing bread with all that pasta. The salmon is a very filling meal that's also lower in carbs if you want to make sure you can fully enjoy the bread before the meal.

(Bonus: If you're looking for some extra fiber or a starter, go with the soup. The minestrone is your best option.)

Outback Steakhouse

Outback Center-Cut Sirloin (6 oz.) + Homestyle Mashed Potatoes

The sirloin cut gives you room to roam. It's not always easy to find mashed potatoes you can enjoy at a restaurant, but this combination makes it all work.

AB Favorite: Victoria's Filet Mignon (8 oz.) + Bread (half the butter)

Ordering the filet will always give you one of the leanest and most tender cuts of meat. It provides the protein and fat to keep you satisfied, and the bread (which has 4 grams of fiber) will ensure you stay full.

Asian Salad with Ahi Tuna

Probably the most underrated item on the menu, with protein, fiber, veggies, and tons of flavor. And it's lower in carbs and fat, which gives you one more reason to enjoy the bread.

Panda Express

Teriyaki Chicken

For fast-food, the majority of Panda Express's chicken meals do a good job of being higher in protein and lower in carbs and fats. But most dishes have very little fiber, and that's where the Teriyaki Chicken stands out.

String Bean Chicken Breast

This dish is the lowest in calories and fat out of all of Panda Express's chicken and chicken breast entrees. Thanks to the string beans, it also has the highest amount of fiber of anything on the menu.

Black Pepper Angus Steak

If you're going to go the steak route, this is your best bet. It's surprisingly filling considering the entire meal is only 170 calories.

Panera Bread

Avocado, Egg White & Spinach on Sprouted Grain Bagel Flat

Proof that bagels can be the breakfast of champions. The sprouted grains add fiber, the eggs bring protein, avocado adds creamy healthy fats, and they sneak in the spinach because you won't even taste it.

Green Goddess Cobb with Chicken (half order, double the chicken)

With a mix of greens (arugula, romaine, kale, and radicchio) the Green Goddess Cobb is a good choice. The double chicken gives you 37 grams of protein with the indulgence of some bacon, and hits the spot with fiber. The green goddess dressing works as long as you add it per the guidelines, but other options that are less caloric include balsamic vinaigrette or olive oil and lemon juice.

Turkey Sandwich + Avocado *or* Bacon (half sandwich)

Panera's turkey options tend to be your best bet, as they give you more room to add on a double portion of protein to leave you extra satisfied. On this sandwich, you'll have to choose whether you'd rather add bacon or avocado, but—ideally—not both.

Bonus: Turkey Chili with Beans (bowl)

Don't sleep on the chili. Typically a side, chili tends to be loaded with protein, fiber, and more vegetables than you realize. It's the perfect hunger-stopper.

Papa John's

Stick with the pizza rules (see page 145) and enjoy.

Pizza Hut

Same guidelines as Domino's. Limit the number of slices. If you want an extra slice, opt for the thin crust.

Popeyes Louisiana Kitchen

Five-Piece Blackened Handcrafted Tenders + Small Fries

This non-breaded option is almost all protein. That means you have room for a side of fries, which also packs a small dose of fiber to round out the meal.

Loaded Chicken Wrap

Enjoy po'boy flavor without the pitfalls of the other wraps on the Popeyes menu. The red beans amp up the fiber content, making this wrap more filling.

Bonafide Chicken Leg (x 2) + Corn on the Cob and Green Beans

Grab two chicken legs, add in the green beans and corn on the cob, and you're enjoying a trifecta of Southern cooking while still applying the tools of a complete meal.

Qdoba Mexican Eats

Qdoba is beloved because—like other fast-casual restaurants—they allow you to build your own creation. Here's what you need to know to navigate the menu to your needs.

Tortilla Option

Opt for two 5.5-inch tortillas instead of one 10-inch tortilla. Don't ask me why (it involves math), but the 10-inch tortilla has three times as many carbs and calories. If you're getting the tortillas, add the following:

Protein: Any one source

For carb-focused plus-one: Protein + rice or beans + guac or sour cream or cheese

For fat-focused plus-one: protein + two of the following: guac or sour cream or cheese

Bowl Option

For carb-focused plus-one: Protein + rice and beans + guac or sour cream or cheese

For fat-focused plus-one: Protein + rice or beans + two of the following: guac or sour cream or cheese

Raising Cane's Chicken Fingers

If you find yourself at Raising Cane's, you're in for some really good chicken. You also have a very limited menu, without much room to roam. If you're going to prevent yourself from going full bliss meal (and, let's be honest, this is the type of place where it makes sense to do so), you really only have one option.

Chicken Fingers (x3)

Order the chicken fingers and limit yourself to just three of them. It's that simple. If you want the sauce, follow the rules and don't go crazy.

Red Lobster

Sirloin Steak (7 oz.) + Baked Potato

When in doubt, the sirloin is usually a safe choice for a great source of protein without loading up on too much fat, and it has almost no carbs. The baked potato adds carbs and fiber to round out your meal.

AD's Favorite: Garlic Shrimp Skewers + Broccoli

One of the more flavorful dishes if you enjoy seafood. And it's low enough in calories that if you're feeling hungry, you can easily add another skewer without a worry.

Rainbow Trout + Baked Potato

Trout is similar to salmon, but it has a little less fat and fewer calories while still being loaded with protein. The combination of fish and potatoes is a satisfying meal.

Red Robin

The Keep It Simple Veggie Burger
I'm not typically a veggie burger type of person, but this one is pretty good because of its unique quinoa-veggie blend. It's flavorful, and—as you might expect—packs more fiber to keep you feeling full.

Ensenada Chicken Platter
Take a couple of ancho-grilled chicken breasts, combine them with salsa, add a side salad and veggies, and you have a winning meal.

AB Favorite: Red's Chili Chili (cup or bowl)
Chili is still undefeated. Another appearance on the list because this dish, once again, strikes a great balance for protein, fiber, fat, and flavor.

Simply Grilled Chicken Sandwich
I almost left this off the list. Not because it doesn't meet the criteria (it does, and has some of the highest fiber content on this list), but because you've probably sensed that most grilled chicken sandwiches are a great option. But I couldn't leave it off because it's pretty good and definitely better than other chicken sandwiches on the list (looking at you, Mc-Donald's).

Sonic Drive-In

The Classic Grilled Chicken Sandwich (no mayo) + Kids' Fries
You can eat it as is or you can ask for no mayo and replace it with kids' fries, and you'll walk away more satisfied.

Grilled Chicken Wrap
While other protein options on the menu tend to be high in fat, this grilled chicken wrap provides a lean source of protein with 30 grams and less than 5 grams of saturated fat. Ask for the light ranch dressing and follow the sauce guidelines.

Sonic's Jr. Burger

Like the other popular fast-food restaurants, if you're looking for a burger, your best bet is the junior size. It's low enough in calories that you can add one additional choice of bacon, cheese, avocado, slaw, or chili.

Starbucks

Turkey Bacon, Cheddar & Egg White Sandwich

As delicious as it is classic! It's hard to beat the combo of eggs and meat. Throw them on a sandwich and it's a great way to start your day or power through the afternoon.

AB Favorite: Egg White & Roasted Red Pepper Egg Bites

I lived off these things in airports. Almost every airport has a Starbucks, and these quick, easy, and delicious bites are great as a snack or meal.

Grilled Chicken and Hummus Protein Box

Some premade boxes are glorified danger-zone foods that do little to fill you up with anything but calories and sugar. That's not the case with this box, which gets bonus points for the 7 grams of fiber per serving.

Subway

Oven Roasted Turkey (six inch)

This sandwich is a grand example of a balanced meal with a carb focus. At 260 calories, Subway's Oven Roasted Turkey contains very low fat, the perfect hit of lean protein, and enough fiber to support fullness. And you can sneak in as many extra veggies as you want.

Sweet Onion Chicken Teriyaki (six inch)

Usually, anything with the words "sweet" feels like it needs to be avoided. But that isn't the case with this sandwich. Even though the teriyaki has some sugar, it's balanced out by the comparatively higher amounts of fiber and protein.

Black Forest Ham Bowls

Many of the bowl options at Subway are not ideal, but the Black Forest Ham is an exception. Even when you add dressing, you're still hitting all the marks on your macros.

Taco Bell

Bean Burrito *or* Chicken/Steak Burrito Supreme

Beans are an underrated example of Tool #2 because they're loaded with protein and fiber that will help fill you up. The bean burrito gets most of its protein from the beans and cheese, or you can opt for the steak or chicken option.

Chicken Soft Taco (x2)

With 160 calories per taco, this option is low in fat and carbs, which means you can easily order two of them without a second thought.

Power Bowl

Bowls are a great option because they put you in control of your plus-one options. Without the tortilla, you can choose more rice and beans (carbs) or lean into more guac and sour cream (fat). Just don't forget the sauce rule for the avocado ranch.

Texas Roadhouse

Sirloin (6 oz.) + Buttered Corn

The steaks at Texas Roadhouse all come with smother options. Pass on those and go with the buttered corn, which tastes better and adds the fiber that you're missing.

Green Chile Chicken

With the exception of Sierra Chicken Pasta and Country Fried Chicken, almost all of the chicken dinners are good options. The best of the options is the Green Chile Chicken, which balances moderate amounts of fat and carbs and gives a good boost of fiber.

Bowl of Texas Red Chili with Beans

You've heard it before, but chili is generally one of the best choices when eating out. Sometimes restaurants replace the good stuff with extra (unnecessary) oils, and that's the case in the non-bean version of this chili (which has more fat and calories). So go for the bean version and get more than 30 grams of protein and 6 grams of fiber.

Wendy's

Apple Pecan Salad

Slightly on the higher side for fat, but this salad has nearly 40 grams of protein, 5 grams of fiber, and a mix of fruits and vegetables.

Grilled Chicken Sandwich *or* Grilled Chicken Wrap

At most fast-food burger places, you'll find the chicken sandwiches or wraps fall within the guidelines of providing moderate protein, carbs, and fats.

Junior Cheeseburger Deluxe or the Junior Burger

The easiest way to enjoy a Wendy's burger is to downsize. Either of these options gives you all the flavor and enjoyment by simply reducing the portion of the meal.

Whataburger

Whataburger Jr. (double protein) or Bacon and Cheese Whataburger Jr.

If you want a burger, you're pretty limited at Whataburger (assuming you're not enjoying a bliss meal). But you do have options—either of these two junior versions will work, even if they're a little low on the fiber side.

Garden Salad with Grilled Chicken

It's not exciting, but it's by far the most nutritious option on the menu. You're probably not headed to Whataburger for a salad, but if you're short on options, you won't go wrong here.

Grilled Chicken Melt

The ultimate hack at Whataburger? Forget the chicken sandwich with mayo or sauce and go with the melt version. You add more protein and a healthier source of fat with fewer overall calories.

Wingstop

It finally happened. When I built this list, I wanted to create options at all fifty of the most-visited restaurants. I reviewed every entree, made adjustments, and visited each. But this is one of those places where you will just have to go with a no-guilt, bliss-point mentality. It's the only restaurant on the list without options that work with the tools in this book. It's not that you can't eat here (remember, healthy eating is not about good versus bad foods), but the restaurant lacks the options to mix and match to create the right blend of protein, carbs, fat, and fiber that would enable anything here to be consumed more than once per week.

Zaxby's

Finding options that work on this menu was one of the hardest. Any of the three options below will get the job done, but most items on the menu are all high in both carbs and fats, with a significant amount of calories.

The Garden House "Zalad"

Controlling the dressing will make a big difference with this salad. It's a little lower on protein than you'd ideally want, but everything else is there for a good meal.

Grilled Chicken Sandwich

The safety blanket of most restaurants, the grilled chicken sandwich comes through again. This recipe has more fat than any other grilled chicken option at other restaurants, which doesn't leave you much room for sides.

Boneless Wings (x 5)

If you love wings, this is a surprisingly decent option. You're not going to get the preferred amount of fiber, but the protein will help keep you full.

Chapter 11

MAKE YOUR FAVORITE TAKEOUT

JUST BECAUSE YOU CAN'T eat takeout every day, doesn't mean you can't enjoy takeout-style favorites regularly. You can easily re-create the meals you love in your kitchen, which will make it easier to stick to the plan. Remember, you can feel fuller if you don't feel like everything you eat is a "health" food.

The benefit of home cooking is that you control the entire process and can make even the tastiest foods bend to your nutritional needs. The biggest problems tend to be time, resources, confidence in your cooking, and knowing what to make.

These recipes account for all those variables. Best of all? I designed these recipes around the meals you typically need to limit at restaurants. Love pancakes but don't want them to have more than 1,000 calories? No problem. Want homemade desserts? I have options for those too (and no, the brownies won't be made with black beans).

It's time to deepen your love of food by seeing how simple it is to make good food taste great. And, when you don't feel like it, you know that the "real" takeout is always an option.

BREAKFAST

CINNAMON RAISIN FRENCH TOAST STICKS

Makes 4 servings, 16 sticks total
Prep time: 25 minutes

4 slices sprouted grain cinnamon raisin bread (I use Ezekiel 4:9), cut each slice
   into 4 sticks
6 pasture-raised eggs
1 cup liquid egg whites (equivalent of 6 egg whites)
2 cups unsweetened vanilla almond milk
1 teaspoon pure vanilla extract
2 scoops whey or plant protein powder
2 tablespoons butter, plus more for greasing pan
3 teaspoons ground cinnamon
2 tablespoons unfiltered raw honey
2 crisp apples, cored, peeled, and very thinly sliced

1. Breathe, because French toast sticks are exciting.
2. Place the bread sticks in a bowl or spread them on a 9 x 13–inch or 10 x 15–inch Pyrex dish.

(cont.)

3. In a large bowl, combine the eggs, egg whites, almond milk, vanilla, and protein powder. Whisk until smooth. Pour the liquid mixture all over the bread and set it aside to soak while you cook the apples.

4. In a medium saucepan over medium heat, combine the butter, cinnamon, honey, and sliced apples. Cook until the apples soften, about three to four minutes, stirring often.

5. Heat a large skillet over medium-high heat. Lay the bread strips in the pan to cover the bottom evenly, top with the apples, and cook for four to five minutes per side, until the toast strips are lightly brown and the apples are crisp on top.

6. Let cool for five to ten minutes before serving.

CHAI PROTEIN SHAKE WITH MACA POWDER

Makes 1 serving
Prep time: 3 to 5 minutes

1 cup unsweetened vanilla almond milk
1 scoop vanilla whey or plant protein powder
¼ cup plain full-fat Greek or Skyr yogurt
1 teaspoon vanilla chai maca powder (I use Gaia Herbs)
1 teaspoon unfiltered raw honey
1 tablespoon all-natural almond butter
1 banana, frozen
Handful of ice cubes
Ground cinnamon, for garnish

1. Combine the almond milk, protein powder, yogurt, maca powder, honey, almond butter, banana, and ice cubes in a high-powered blender. Pulse until smooth.

2. Garnish with cinnamon and enjoy.

OMELET MUFFINS

Makes 3-4 servings, 12 muffins total
Prep time: 40 minutes

Non-stick oil spray
1 cup liquid egg whites
6 pasture-raised eggs
2 cups chopped spinach or baby spinach
⅓ cup thinly sliced yellow onion
½ cup small-diced portobello mushroom
2 uncured, nitrate-free turkey bacon slices, diced small
¼ teaspoon ground black pepper
½ teaspoon Himalayan sea salt
½ teaspoon garlic powder
6 tablespoons grated Parmesan cheese

1. Preheat the oven to 350°F. Line a muffin pan with twelve paper or silicone baking cups. Spray the cups with the non-stick spray.
2. In a medium bowl, whisk the egg whites and eggs until combined. In a large bowl, combine the spinach, onion, mushrooms, bacon, pepper, salt, and garlic powder. Mix in the egg mixture.
3. Use a spoon to divide the batter among the cups, filling each three-quarters full. (The muffins will puff up a little while they're cooking.) Sprinkle ½ tablespoon Parmesan on top of each one.
4. Bake for 25 to 30 minutes, until the muffins are cooked through (a thin knife inserted into a muffin will come out clean) and the Parmesan has slightly browned on top.
5. Let cool for five to ten minutes. Enjoy warm, or pack in Tupperware containers for an easy, grab-and-go breakfast bite. These can last up to one week in an airtight container in the fridge.

SAUSAGE BREAKFAST PITA

Makes 1 serving
Prep time: 10 minutes

½ tablespoon extra-virgin olive oil
¼ cup small-diced yellow onion
1 precooked chicken sausage, small diced
1 cup packed baby spinach
½ cup liquid egg whites
¼ teaspoon garlic powder
Sea salt and ground black pepper, to taste
1 tablespoon shredded Parmesan cheese
1 pita

1. In a medium skillet over medium heat, heat the oil and add the onion and sausage. Stir to combine, then let sausage edges brown and the onions caramelize for a few minutes. Add the spinach, stir, and cook until it's wilted. Add the egg whites and scramble to your liking. Season with the garlic powder, sea salt, and pepper. Add the Parmesan and stir.
2. Stuff the scramble into the pita. It doesn't have to be pretty. Pray the pita doesn't break. If it does, grab a fork. Be civilized. Eat.

BACON AND DATE PROTEIN PANCAKES

Makes 2 servings, 4 pancakes total
Prep time: 25 minutes

4 slices uncured, nitrate-free turkey bacon
1 cup old-fashioned rolled oats
1 teaspoon baking powder
1 scoop whey or plant protein powder
¼ teaspoon ground cinnamon
2 pasture-raised eggs
1 cup liquid egg whites
½ cup milk or plant milk of your choice
½ teaspoon pure vanilla extract
2 tablespoons butter
5 dates, pitted and finely chopped
2 tablespoons pure maple syrup

1. In a small sauté pan on medium-high heat, cook the turkey bacon until crispy, three to four minutes per side. Remove from the pan, crumble into small bits, and set aside.
2. Combine the oats, baking powder, protein powder, and cinnamon in a blender or food processor. Pulse until the oats are the texture of flour. Set aside.
3. In a medium bowl, whisk the eggs, egg whites, milk, and vanilla. Slowly mix the dry ingredients into the wet ingredients until just combined, taking care not to overmix.
4. Add 1 teaspoon of the butter to the pan and melt it over medium-high heat. Pour in ¼ cup of the pancake batter. Sprinkle with one-sixth of the chopped dates and sprinkle one-sixth of the crumbled bacon on top. When the top of the pancake begins to bubble, about three minutes, it's ready to flip. Repeat to cook the other side for two or three minutes, then plate the pancake.
5. Repeat with the remaining batter to make five more pancakes, using a bit more butter as needed.
6. To cut down on the sugar in the syrup, mix it with 2 tablespoons water and 1 teaspoon of the butter in a small bowl. Heat in the microwave for ten seconds, stir, and pour over the pancakes. Enjoy immediately.

PEANUT BUTTER–BANANA OVERNIGHT OATS

Makes 1 serving
Prep time: 5 minutes

¼ cup old-fashioned rolled oats
¾ cup unsweetened vanilla almond milk
1 tablespoon chia seeds
1 tablespoon creamy peanut butter
1 tablespoon peanut butter powder
½ banana, cut into small chunks
¼ cup nonfat plain Greek yogurt
1 scoop whey or plant protein powder

1. Combine all the ingredients in a bowl or mason jar and mix well.
2. Cover and refrigerate overnight. (Technically, it needs to chill for two and a half to three hours before the oats achieve a good texture.)
3. Eat the next day or two and a half to three hours later, and wonder why you ever doubted me. Yes, it's that good. So good, in fact, you might make this every day.

VEGGIE EGG SANDWICH

Makes 1 serving
Prep time: 20 minutes

Oil spray
2 cups roughly chopped spinach
3 pasture-raised eggs
1 large portobello mushroom cap, cut into small dice
1 tablespoon goat cheese
2 slices high-fiber bread (more than 3 grams of fiber per slice)

1. Spray the pan and warm it over medium-high heat.
2. Add the spinach and sauté for about two minutes, until just wilted. Add the eggs, mushrooms, and goat cheese and scramble until the eggs are cooked to your liking.
3. Sandwich the cooked ingredients in the bread. Enjoy!

CREAMY STRAWBERRY SMOOTHIE

Makes 1 serving
Prep time: 5 minutes

1 cup frozen strawberries
¼ cup old-fashioned rolled oats
1 scoop vanilla whey or plant protein powder
2 tablespoons low-fat plain Greek yogurt
1 cup unsweetened vanilla almond milk

1. Combine all the ingredients in a blender and blend until smooth.
2. Drink, and wonder why you ever stopped having strawberry milk.

CHOCOLATE-BANANA–PEANUT BUTTER PROTEIN SMOOTHIE

Makes 1 serving
Prep time: 5 minutes

2 handfuls ice cubes
1 cup dairy milk or plant milk of your choice
1 banana
1 scoop chocolate whey or plant protein powder
1 tablespoon peanut butter
½ cup cauliflower florets (fresh or frozen)

More blender magic. Combine all the ingredients and press the miracle button.
Enjoy!

MOCHA PROTEIN SHAKE

Makes 1 serving
Prep time: 5 minutes

1 cup iced black coffee
½ frozen large banana
2 handfuls ice cubes
1 scoop chocolate whey or plant protein powder
1 tablespoon all-natural almond butter

1. If we don't provide instructions for a protein shake, does it even exist?
2. We hope you figured it out and are drinking this thing. It's insanely good.

PEACHES AND GREENS SMOOTHIE BOWL

Makes 1 serving
Prep time: 5 minutes

1 small handful baby spinach
½ cup plain low-fat Greek yogurt
½ cup unsweetened vanilla almond milk
1 cup frozen peach slices (or 1 peach, pitted and sliced)
1 handful ice
1 scoop unflavored whey or plant protein powder
1 teaspoon chia seeds
½ teaspoon pure vanilla extract
1 handful granola

1. In a blender, combine the spinach, yogurt, almond milk, peach slices, ice, protein powder, chia seeds, and vanilla.
2. Serve in a bowl and top with the granola.

LUNCH

HIGH-PROTEIN GRILLED CHEESE

Makes 1 serving
Prep time: 10 minutes

1 tablespoon butter
2 thick slices of bread (sourdough recommended)
¼ cup shredded Parmesan (about one handful)
1 slice fat-free cheddar cheese
1 slice low-fat mozzarella
1 slice provolone

1. Realize you get to eat grilled cheese on a diet plan!
2. Heat a skillet over medium heat.
3. Butter one side of each piece of bread with ½ tablespoon butter.
4. Place the bread buttered side down in the skillet. Add the Parmesan and cheddar to one slice and the mozzarella and provolone to the other.
5. Let cook for three to four minutes, until the cheese is melting and the bread is lightly toasted, then close the sandwich with the cheeses inside. Cook for one minute. Flip the sandwich and cook for one to two more minutes, until nice and toasted.
6. Serve, beware of the hot cheese, and good luck eating just one of these. But seriously, you'll feel full—and stay full—once it hits.

BUFFALO CHICKEN QUESADILLA

Makes 4-6 servings, 1 quesadilla per serving
Prep time: 15 minutes

1 rotisserie chicken
2 cups buffalo sauce (Frank's RedHot works great)
1 teaspoon garlic powder
1 teaspoon chili powder
One 5-inch flourless tortilla per serving
¼ avocado, sliced thin

1. Use a fork to pull the meat from the rotisserie chicken. Place it in a medium bowl. Discard the bones and skin.
2. In a medium saucepan, combine the chicken, buffalo sauce, garlic powder, and chili powder. Set the pan over low heat and heat through, stirring occasionally.
3. Heat a large cast-iron (or other) skillet over medium-high heat.
4. Place 1 tortilla in the skillet and spread ½ cup of the shredded chicken on top, leaving about 1 inch around the edges. Top with the avocado slices, then the other tortilla. Toast each side for about five minutes, until the cheese melts and the tortilla turns a golden brown. Use a large spatula to flip. (You can also bake in the toaster oven on high, or in a conventional oven on 425°F for about five to eight minutes.) Repeat to make the rest of the quesadillas.
5. Let cool, then cut into triangles. A pizza cutter works well if you have one!
6. Save any remaining shredded chicken for the week's lunches as a protein salad topper or for a sandwich or wrap. It's great in the Mediterranean Rotisserie Pita on page 187.

HONEY MUSTARD CHICKEN BLT WRAP

Makes 6 wraps
Prep time: 20 minutes

6 slices uncured, nitrate-free bacon
1 rotisserie chicken, meat removed and shredded, or two 12.5-ounce cans
   chicken breast
⅓ cup full-fat plain Greek yogurt
⅓ cup Dijon mustard
¼ cup unfiltered raw honey
Himalayan salt, to taste
Ground black pepper, to taste
Garlic powder, to taste
Six 8-inch sprouted grain wraps
2 cups mixed greens
½ tomato, cut into six thin slices

1. In a large skillet over medium-high heat, cook the turkey bacon until crispy,
   about five minutes. Remove from the pan, crumble into small bits, and set
   aside.
2. Place the chicken in a medium bowl and break up the pieces with a fork. Add
   the yogurt, mustard, honey, salt, pepper, garlic powder, and crumbled bacon.
   Mix well to combine.
3. Heat a wrap in a warm oven or in the microwave for 10 to 20 seconds to
   soften. Add approximately ⅙ of the chicken salad to one corner of the wrap.
   Add ⅓ cup of the mixed greens and a tomato slice. Roll up and repeat to
   make the rest of the wraps. Enjoy!

TURKEY TACOS

Makes 3-4 servings, 6-8 tacos total
Prep time: 20 minutes

1 tablespoon unrefined, cold-pressed coconut oil
1 thinly sliced yellow onion
1 thinly sliced red bell pepper
1 thinly sliced yellow bell pepper
1 pound lean ground turkey
1 tablespoon chili powder
1 teaspoon smoked paprika
1 teaspoon garlic powder
1 teaspoon Himalayan salt
½ teaspoon cayenne
Six to eight 7-inch grain-free tortillas

Taco toppings
1 cup defrosted frozen corn
1 avocado, sliced
Salsa, optional
Lettuce or spinach, finely chopped

1. In a large skillet over medium-high heat, melt the coconut oil. Add the onions and peppers and sauté until softened, about five minutes. Add the ground turkey, break into pieces, and cook until the turkey starts to brown. Add the spices and stir. Reduce the heat to medium-low and cover. Cook until the turkey is no longer pink, about five to ten minutes.
2. Meanwhile, prepare the toppings in small serving bowls. Or don't. If you're eating for one, you can just make the tacos and eat them plain.
3. Heat the tortillas for five to ten seconds in the microwave and divide the turkey mixture and taco toppings among them as desired. Enjoy immediately!

CHICKEN NOODLE SOUP

Makes 1 large pot of soup, 1 cup per serving
Prep time: 60 minutes

6 boneless skinless chicken breasts, cut into 1-inch cubes
½ teaspoon Himalayan or iodized sea salt, plus more to taste
½ teaspoon ground black pepper, plus more to taste
2 tablespoons extra-virgin olive oil
3 minced garlic cloves
1 small diced yellow onion
2 large carrots, peeled and cut into small dice
2 small diced celery stalks
10 trimmed and halved Brussels sprouts
6 cups low-sodium organic chicken stock
2 cups pasta shells
½ cup frozen peas
2 bay leaves
1 teaspoon dried thyme

1. Preheat the oven to 375°F.
2. Season the chicken with the salt and pepper. Spread it in a 7 x 11-inch Pyrex or other pan, cover with aluminum foil, and bake for 25 to 30 minutes, until cooked through.
3. In a large pot over medium heat, heat the olive oil. Add the garlic and onion and sauté for three to five minutes, until golden, then add the carrots, celery, and Brussels sprouts. Cook for five to ten minutes, until the vegetables are softened, stirring occasionally.
4. Add the chicken stock, cover the pot, turn up the heat, and bring to a boil. Add the pasta shells, peas, bay leaves, thyme, and salt and pepper to taste. Cook about five minutes, until the pasta is cooked (be careful, it gets mushy fast).
5. Lower the heat, add the chicken, and stir. Simmer until the chicken is heated through, one to two minutes.
6. Serve hot and enjoy! Save the soup in an airtight container in the fridge for up to five days or the freezer for up to a month.

SHRIMP WRAPS

Makes 1 serving, 2 wraps total
Prep time: 5 minutes

Two medium size (7-inch) flour tortillas
2 handfuls pre-cooked shrimp (21/25 or 26/30 count work great)
Hot sauce and/or sliced avocado (optional)

1. Lay out the tortillas.
2. If you want, you can heat the shrimp on a skillet, microwave, or air fryer. It's up to you, but this is designed to be a quick, easy, delicious meal. Divide the shrimp between the two tortillas.
3. Top with hot sauce and/or avocado slices, if using, and wrap up each tortilla. Easy as 1–2–3.

SLOW-COOKER BUTTERNUT SQUASH SOUP

Makes about 4 cups, 1 cup per serving
Prep time: 3 to 4 hours on low; 5 to 6 hours on high; 15 minutes active

2 small butternut squash, peeled, seeded, and cut into ½-inch cubes (about 3 cups of cubed butternut squash)
1 large sweet potato, peeled and cut into ½-inch cubes
4 garlic cloves
2 cups low-sodium chicken or vegetable broth
½ teaspoon Himalayan salt
1 teaspoon ground turmeric
½ teaspoon smoked paprika
¼ teaspoon cayenne
1 teaspoon finely grated fresh ginger (or ½ teaspoon ground ginger)
Pumpkin seeds, to top (toasted or raw)
Sliced basil, to top
Cooked protein of your choice (a great use for leftovers)

1. Combine the butternut squash, sweet potato, garlic, and broth in a slow cooker, set the cooker to low, and cook about five to six hours, until softened. Let cool a bit.
2. Working in batches as needed, pour the mixture into a blender and add the salt, turmeric, paprika, cayenne, and ginger. Blend to your desired consistency: two minutes for smooth, 30 seconds of short pulses for chunky.

3. Garnish with the pumpkin seeds and sliced basil. Serve with the protein of your choice.

MEDITERRANEAN ROTISSERIE PITA

Makes 1 serving
Prep time: 10 minutes

1 whole wheat pita
1½ tablespoons full fat Greek yogurt
1½ tablespoons hummus
1 tablespoon crumbled feta cheese
1 cup shredded rotisserie chicken (or leftover slow-cooked chicken from Buffalo Chicken Quesadilla, page 182)
2 or 3 thinly sliced grape tomatoes
10 thin cucumber slices
3 sliced black olives
Sea salt, to taste
Ground black pepper, to taste

1. If desired, heat the pita in a dry skillet over medium heat for one to two minutes or in the microwave for 10 to 20 seconds.
2. Spread the yogurt over half of the pita and the hummus over the other half. Top with the crumbled feta. On one half of the pita, pile the chicken, tomatoes, cucumber, and olives.
3. Sprinkle with salt and pepper to taste. Fold over and enjoy!

STEAK SANDWICH

Makes 1 serving
Prep time: 15 minutes

4 to 6 ounces lean steak (sirloin), cut into ¼-inch slices
Salt, to taste
Ground black pepper, to taste
½ tablespoon extra-virgin olive oil or butter
½ thinly sliced small yellow onion
2 slices of your favorite bread or hoagie (with more than 4 grams of fiber)

(cont.)

1. Season the steak with salt and pepper.
2. Warm the olive oil or butter in a skillet over medium-high heat. Add the onions. Stir occasionally until they start to brown, approximately five minutes.
3. Move the onions to the side of the pan and add the steak. Cook it to the desired doneness (medium will be about three to four minutes per side).
4. Place the steak and onions on the bread. Do what you were born to do and enjoy the meal.

AVOCADO TUNA SALAD

Makes 1 serving
Prep time: 10 minutes

2 tablespoons almond slivers
One 5-ounce can albacore tuna
½ ripe avocado, mashed
½ lemon, juiced
½ teaspoon mustard powder
¼ teaspoon garlic powder
Dash of Himalayan sea salt
Dash of ground black pepper
Bed of lettuce *or* 1 whole-grain pita *or* 8 whole-grain crackers

1. Toast the almonds in a dry skillet over low heat for a few minutes, until lightly browned, stirring often and watching carefully so they don't burn.
2. Rinse the tuna under cold running water for about a minute. This helps to clean out some of the preservatives used in canning and will help decrease that fishy smell and taste.
3. In a large bowl, combine tuna, avocado, lemon juice, mustard, garlic, salt and pepper. Using a large fork, break up the chunks of tuna and mix evenly.
4. Top with the toasted almond slivers for an added texture and nice crunchy bite.
5. Enjoy on a bed of lettuce, stuffed into a pita, or with crackers on the side.

DINNER

STEAK STIR-FRY

Makes 4 servings
Prep time: 20 minutes

1 pound flank steak, cut into ¼-inch slices
Sea salt, to taste
Ground black pepper, to taste
½ tablespoon extra-virgin olive oil
2 garlic cloves, minced
2 handfuls spinach
1 broccoli head, cut into florets
1 finely chopped medium yellow onion
8 ounces snow peas
1 tablespoon soy sauce
1 to 2 tablespoons sriracha

1. Season the steak with a good amount of salt and pepper, or to taste.
2. Heat the oil in a large nonstick or cast-iron skillet over medium-high heat.

(cont.)

Add the garlic and sauté until just lightly browned, 30 to 60 seconds. Add the steak and cook, stirring occasionally, for three to five minutes per side, to your desired doneness. Transfer to a plate and set aside.

3. Add the spinach, broccoli, and onion to the skillet and sauté for about three minutes on medium-high heat, until the vegetables start to soften. Stir in the snow peas and sauté for two minutes.

4. Reduce the heat to low, return the steak to the skillet, add the soy sauce and sriracha to taste, and stir until combined and heated through.

5. Plate it. Eat it.

PROTEIN NACHOS

Makes 4 servings, about 40 loaded nachos total
Prep time: 20 minutes

1 tablespoon extra-virgin olive oil or unrefined, cold-pressed coconut oil
1 pound ground beef or turkey (at least 90% lean)
1 teaspoon sea salt
1 teaspoon chili powder
One 12-ounce can black beans, rinsed and drained
1 cup frozen or canned corn, rinsed and drained
5 ounces tortilla chips (about 45 chips)
1 thinly sliced jalapeño pepper
3 diced scallions
⅓ cup shredded cheese of your choice (cheddar, mozzarella, or pepper Jack all work great)
1 diced avocado

1. In a large skillet over medium-high heat, heat the oil. Add the ground meat and cook, stirring and breaking the meat up as it cooks, until the meat is no longer pink and has started to brown, about ten minutes. Season with the salt and chili powder, stir, and cook for about five minutes, until cooked through.

2. Preheat the oven to 425°F.

3. Combine the beans and corn in a microwave-safe bowl and microwave until heated through, 30 to 60 seconds.

4. Lay the chips in a single layer on a large sheet pan. Top with the meat, then with the black beans and corn. Add the jalapeño, scallions, and cheese.

5. Bake for five minutes, until the cheese melts on top.

6. Top with diced avocado and feast.

TACOS (STEAK, FISH, CHICKEN, OR SHRIMP)

Makes 4 servings
Prep time: 25 minutes

1 pound protein of your choice, such as steak, chicken, fish, or shrimp (if using steak or chicken, thinly slice; if using fish, cut into chunks; if using shrimp, peel entirely and cut in half if large)

½ teaspoon cayenne pepper

1 tablespoon chili powder

1 teaspoon garlic powder

2 tablespoons unrefined avocado oil

1 thinly sliced red onion

3 thinly sliced bell peppers, any color

1 teaspoon sea salt

8 hard corn taco shells

⅓ cup shredded cheese (cheddar or pepper jack)

1 thinly sliced avocado

2 cups shredded lettuce

½ cup chopped cilantro

1. Season the protein with the cayenne, chili, and garlic.
2. Heat a large skillet over medium-high heat and add the oil. Add the onions and peppers. Cook until the peppers start to sizzle and soften, three to five minutes.
3. Add the protein to the peppers, season with the salt, and cook to your desired doneness.
4. Try to stand up your taco shells. (Good luck.)
5. Divide the mixture among the taco shells. Top with cheese, avocado, lettuce, and cilantro, and serve.

CAPRESE BISON BURGERS

Makes 4 servings
Prep time: 20 minutes

Bison Burgers
  1 pound ground bison (ideally 90% lean)
  1 teaspoon sea salt
  1 teaspoon ground black pepper
  2 tablespoons extra-virgin olive oil
  4 sprouted-grain or whole wheat buns
  1 cup mixed greens, packed
  1 thinly sliced tomato
  One 4-ounce mozzarella ball, cut into four slices

Balsamic Mustard Spread
  2 tablespoons Dijon mustard
  1 teaspoon extra-virgin olive oil
  1 tablespoon balsamic vinegar
  Salt, to taste
  Ground black pepper, to taste

1. In a medium bowl, mix the ground bison, salt, and pepper. Divide the mixture into four burger patties, making them about ½-inch wider than your buns, and gently press an indent in the center with your thumb.
2. Set a large skillet over medium heat and grease it lightly with olive oil. Add the burger patties and cook them for about five minutes per side, until lightly browned. The interior should be light pink, but cook them longer if you want your burgers more cooked through.
3. While the burgers cook, take a picture and tag @bornfitness on Instagram. Why? Because I love burgers and seeing people enjoy them while "on a diet" will bring more joy to the world. After you snap your picture, stir the mustard spread ingredients together in a small bowl. Set aside.
4. Spread the balsamic mustard spread on the bottom half of each bun. Top each with ¼ cup mixed greens, burger patty, tomato slice, mozzarella slice, and the top bun.
5. It's burger time.

PEANUT PAD THAI AND SHRIMP

Makes 2 servings
Prep time: 30 minutes

Pad Thai
    2 ounces uncooked rice noodles
    2 tablespoons sesame or avocado oil
    2 minced garlic cloves
    1 teaspoon minced fresh ginger (or ½ teaspoon ground ginger)
    1 thinly sliced red bell pepper
    1 julienned large carrot
    12 uncooked fresh or thawed frozen jumbo shrimp (peeled, tails removed)
    ½ cup mung bean sprouts

Peanut Sauce
    1 tablespoon water
    1 tablespoon smooth or crunchy all-natural peanut butter
    1 teaspoon sriracha
    1 tablespoon low-sodium soy sauce or liquid aminos
    1 tablespoon apple cider vinegar
    ½ tablespoon unfiltered raw honey
    ½ teaspoon chili powder

Garnish
    ½ lime, cut into wedges
    Chopped fresh cilantro
    ¼ cup roughly chopped peanuts

1. Cook the noodles until soft according to the package directions.
2. Meanwhile, combine the peanut sauce ingredients and whisk until smooth.
3. In a large skillet or wok, combine the oil, garlic, and ginger. Sauté on medium-high heat for about one minute (don't let the garlic burn), then add the bell peppers, carrots, and shrimp. Stir fry for about three minutes, until the shrimp is pink all the way through but not overcooked.
4. Remove from the heat and add the noodles, mung beans, and peanut sauce. Toss together to fully coat.
5. Divide between two bowls and garnish with lime wedges, cilantro, and peanuts. Serve warm.

NAKED CHICKEN TENDERS

Makes 2 to 3 servings
Prep time: 25 minutes

1 pound chicken breasts
2 tablespoons extra-virgin olive oil
2 tablespoons sea salt
2 tablespoons ground black pepper
2 tablespoons garlic powder
1 tablespoon cayenne
1 tablespoon onion powder
2 tablespoons of your favorite BBQ sauce

1. Rub the chicken breasts with the olive oil and season with the salt, pepper, garlic powder, cayenne, and onion powder. Let sit for five minutes.
2. Heat a large skillet over medium-high heat and add the chicken in a single layer. Cook for five to seven minutes per side, until the chicken is white inside (at least 165°F). Slice the chicken into strips or cut them into nuggets if you prefer.
3. Pour the BBQ sauce onto your plate (or into a little bowl, if you're fancy). Dip and devour.

CHICKEN BURRITOS

Makes 4 servings
Prep time: 20 minutes

1 tablespoon extra-virgin olive oil
4 chicken breasts (cheat code: use a rotisserie chicken)
1 tablespoon sea salt
1 tablespoon ground black pepper
4 large (10-inch) flour tortillas
One 15.5-ounce can low-sodium kidney beans, drained and rinsed
1 cup frozen corn, thawed and warmed
2 thinly sliced scallions
¼ cup shredded cheese (cheddar is great, but please yourself)
1 cup finely shredded lettuce
1 tomato, diced small
2 teaspoons lime juice

1. In a large skillet over medium-high heat, heat the olive oil. Cut the chicken into small cubes, season the chicken with the salt and pepper, and lay it in the skillet. Cook for five to eight minutes on each side, until cooked through (or just warm up some rotisserie chicken in the microwave).
2. Warm the tortillas in the microwave for 30 to 60 seconds.
3. Divide the chicken, kidney beans, corn, scallions, cheese, lettuce, tomato, and lime juice among the tortillas. Roll up the tortillas burrito-style to enclose the ingredients. Toast everyone at the dinner table and enjoy.

SLOW-COOKER HIGH-PROTEIN SWEET POTATO CHILI

Makes 4 to 6 servings
Prep time: 15 minutes active: 3 to 4 hours on high or 5 to 6 hours on low

3 medium sweet potatoes, cut into ¼-inch dice
One 28-ounce can diced tomatoes
One 10-ounce can tomato sauce
1 large sweet onion, cut into small dice
¼ cup celery, cut into small dice
2 cups water or chicken stock
2 tablespoons chili powder
2 teaspoons ground cumin
2 jalapeño peppers, cut into small dice
2 teaspoons sea salt
1 teaspoon ground black pepper
1 teaspoon cayenne
1 tablespoon garlic powder
2 teaspoons smoked paprika
1 teaspoon onion powder
One 15-ounce can black beans, drained and rinsed
One 15-ounce can kidney beans, drained and rinsed
1 tablespoon unrefined, cold-pressed coconut oil
1 pound ground turkey or grass-fed beef (90% lean or leaner)
½ pound boneless, skinless chicken breast, cut into 1-inch cubes
¼ thinly sliced avocado
2 thinly sliced scallions

1. In a slow cooker, combine the sweet potatoes, tomatoes, tomato sauce, onion, celery, water, chili powder, cumin, jalapeños, salt, black pepper, cayenne, garlic powder, smoked paprika, onion powder, and beans.
2. Heat the coconut oil in a large skillet over medium-high heat. Add the meat and brown it until almost cooked through, about five minutes, breaking it up in the pan as needed. Add the meat to the slow cooker.
3. In the same pan over medium heat, cook the chicken for five to ten minutes, until you no longer see pink on the outside (it doesn't have to be fully cooked; the slow cooker will do the rest). Add the chicken to the slow cooker and stir to combine.
4. Cook the chili on high for three to four hours or on low for five to six hours. The sweet potatoes should be tender but not mushy.
5. Top with avocado slices and scallions. Eat and be satisfied.

SWEET POTATO MAC-N-CHEESE BITES WITH BACON

Makes 6 servings, 12 muffin-size bites total
Prep time: 60 minutes

Oil spray or muffin liners
4 uncured, nitrate-free bacon slices
One 1-pound sweet potato, peeled and cut into 1-inch cubes
4 tablespoons (½ stick) butter
3 tablespoons all-purpose flour
1 cup whole milk
¼ cup crumbled goat cheese
¾ cup shredded reduced-fat cheddar cheese
1 teaspoon smoked paprika
Sea salt and ground black pepper, to taste
2 cups uncooked small pasta shells
¼ cup shredded Parmigiano-Reggiano

1. Preheat the oven to 400°F. Lightly grease 12 muffin cups or line them with paper liners. Line a sheet pan with parchment paper.

2. Lay the bacon on the prepared sheet pan and bake for 10 to 15 minutes, until crisp. Let cool, crumble, and set aside.

3. Meanwhile, bring water to a boil in a large pot and add the sweet potato chunks. Boil until they can easily be pierced with a fork, about ten minutes. Strain out the sweet potato chunks and place them in a bowl (you'll use the same water for boiling the pasta shells).

4. Mash the sweet potatoes with a fork. Set aside.

5. In a large skillet over medium heat, combine the butter and flour. Cook, whisking, until you have a light golden roux, about five minutes. Remove from the heat and whisk in the milk, continuing to whisk until the mixture is thickened. Slowly add the goat and cheddar cheeses, paprika, salt, and pepper, whisking as the cheeses melt in. Go easy on the salt, as cheese is already salty. When the cheese mixture is smooth, add the mashed sweet potato.

6. Meanwhile, bring the water to a boil again and add the pasta. Start checking for doneness two to three minutes before the package says it should be finished. Do not overcook the pasta; it will become mushy. Reserve ½ cup pasta water and drain out the rest.

7. Add the cooked pasta and ¼ cup of the pasta water to the cheese mixture. Mix thoroughly to combine, stirring in a bit more pasta water to make the texture to your liking.

(cont.)

8. You can easily serve as is now, with each serving sprinkled with bacon and parm. But I love baked mac-n-cheese, so I made this into muffin-size bites. (You can also spread the mixture in a large glass pan and bake at 425°F for about 20 minutes, until you see the top start to brown and crisp.) Add ¼ cup of the mac-n-cheese mix to each muffin cup. Top with the crumbled bacon and a little pinch of Parmigiano-Reggiano. Bake for ten minutes, until golden. Prepare to be obsessed.

FISH FOIL PACKETS

Makes 1 serving, but you'll want to make a lot more
Prep time: 40 minutes

4 ounces fish: salmon, trout, tuna, or other fish of your choice
1½ cups of veggies (pick three or four): sugar snap peas, snow peas, watercress, spinach, pickled baby corn, sliced carrots, bell peppers, mushrooms, broccoli, onion
Fat (pick 1): handful of sliced nuts or ½ avocado
Carb (pick 1): ½ cup uncooked rice or quinoa or 2 slices of bread (if you prefer a fish sandwich)
Sauce: soy, teriyaki, or sriracha

1. Preheat the oven to 400°F.
2. For each serving, place the protein, veggies, and fat in the center of a 10-inch-long foil sheet. Lay a second foil sheet on top and crimp the edges together to create a packet.
3. Place the packets on a sheet pan. Bake for 25 minutes. Open one packet and use a fork to check and make sure the fish is flaky and has lost its translucent, raw appearance. If not, cook for another 5 minutes. Note: Do not open the packets to check them until 25 minutes are up, as you'll let out the steam and slow the cooking process.
4. Meanwhile, cook the rice or quinoa, if using.
5. Open the packets, place on a plate with the rice or quinoa, add your choice of sauce, and feast. Well, maybe wait five minutes—it's gonna be hot.

BAKED FISH AND VEGGIES

Makes 4 servings
Prep time: 35 minutes

> 1 broccoli head, chopped into small florets
> 4 or 5 medium carrots, peeled and sliced into ¼-inch rounds
> 1 small yellow onion, finely chopped
> 2 small sweet potatoes, peeled and diced into small cubes
> 2 tablespoons avocado oil
> Sea salt, to taste
> 12 ounces fresh or flash-frozen fish fillets
> Ground black pepper, to taste

1. Preheat the oven to 400°F. Line two sheet pans with parchment paper.
2. Place the vegetables on one of the prepared sheet pans and top with 1 tablespoon of the oil. Give two or three shakes of salt and pepper and toss to combine. Roast for 15 minutes, until the veggies are softened.
3. While the veggies are roasting, prepare the fish on the second prepared sheet pan. Coat the fillet or fillets with the remaining 1 tablespoon of oil and season with salt and pepper to taste. When the 15-minute timer goes off, set the pan with the fish in the oven.
4. Roast the veggies and fish together for 10 to 12 minutes, until the fish is cooked through and the veggies are nicely roasted. Remove from the oven and feast.

SALADS

TOMATO, CUCUMBER, AVOCADO, AND HERB SALAD

Makes 5 to 6 servings
Prep time: 10 minutes (assuming the protein is already cooked)

2 pints grape tomatoes
½ English cucumber, diced
6 fresh basil leaves or small parsley sprigs, or a mix, finely chopped
½ cup small-diced red onion
3 tablespoons extra-virgin olive oil
1 lemon, juiced
¾ teaspoon sea salt
½ teaspoon ground black pepper
¼ cup crumbled feta cheese
1 avocado, pitted, peeled, and cut into ¼-inch dice
Cooked protein of your choice (such as chicken, fish, or steak)

1. In a large bowl, combine all the ingredients except the feta, avocado, and protein. Toss to mix well. Add the feta and avocado and lightly toss.
2. Serve with your favorite source of protein to make it a complete meal. You can store this salad in an airtight container in the fridge for up to five days. If you plan on making this in bulk and eating throughout the week, I recommend leaving out the olive oil, feta, and avocado until you're ready to eat!

APPLE AND BACON-ROASTED BRUSSELS SPROUTS

Makes 8 servings
Prep time: 50 minutes

> 2 pounds Brussels sprouts, trimmed and halved
> 1 crisp apple (such as Fuji), cored and cut into ½-inch dice
> 3 slices uncured, nitrate-free turkey bacon (feel free to substitute a plant-based version if vegetarian), chopped
> 2 tablespoons avocado oil
> ½ teaspoon garlic powder
> ½ teaspoon Himalayan salt
> ¼ teaspoon ground black pepper
> ¼ cup slivered almonds

1. Preheat the oven to 425°F.
2. In a large bowl, combine the Brussels sprouts, apple, bacon, avocado oil, garlic powder, salt, and pepper. Toss until fully coated.
3. Spread the mixture in an even layer on a sheet pan. Bake for 35 to 40 minutes, until the Brussels sprouts are brown, crisp, and tender.
4. Remove from the oven and sprinkle the almond slivers on top. Bake for five minutes, until the almonds are lightly toasted.
5. Serve warm as a side dish or cold in a packed lunch.

FETA AND CHICKPEA QUINOA SALAD

Makes 4 servings
Prep time: 15 minutes

⅓ cup almond slivers
½ tablespoon extra-virgin olive oil
2 teaspoons minced garlic
2 cups cooked quinoa (from ⅔ cup uncooked quinoa cooked in water or low-sodium chicken broth)
¼ cup sliced sundried tomatoes
½ cup quartered artichoke hearts, canned in water
One 15.5-ounce can chickpeas, drained and rinsed
½ tablespoon butter
2 fresh basil leaves, thinly sliced
Juice from half a lemon
¼ teaspoon Himalayan sea salt
Ground black pepper, to taste
¼ cup crumbled feta cheese, optional
Grilled chicken breasts, for serving, optional

1. In a large skillet over low heat, toast the almond slivers until lightly browned, stirring often, about three minutes. Set aside.
2. In the same skillet over medium heat, heat the olive oil. Add the garlic and cook, stirring often, for about one minute, until golden. Add the quinoa, tomatoes, artichoke hearts, chickpeas, almond slivers, butter, basil, lemon juice, salt, and pepper. Cook, stirring often, for five to ten minutes, to let the flavors develop. Toss in the feta, if using.
3. Serve alone for a light, vegetarian-friendly meal or add a grilled chicken breast to bump up the protein.

TACO SALAD

Makes 2 servings
Prep time: 5 minutes (with pre-cooked protein)

Some recipes aren't really "recipes" but reminders that you can create an amazing meal by combining great ingredients that add the perfect mix of nutrition and flavor. This taco salad is the perfect representation of the "no-recipe recipe." Simply take the ingredients below, toss them in a bowl, and enjoy!

Greens (romaine, kale, or spring mix), chopped
Lean ground turkey, cooked and seasoned with taco seasoning
Black beans, rinsed and drained
Avocado, sliced
Red bell pepper, sliced
Kernels from cooked fresh sweet corn (or warm up frozen corn)
Salsa
Plain Greek yogurt

1. Lay the greens in a bowl or on a plate and assemble the meat, beans, and vegetables on top.
2. Dollop on a spoon of salsa and a spoon of yogurt (this will act as your dressing).
3. Toss and enjoy!

DESSERTS

CINNAMON-APPLE PARFAIT WITH PROTEIN GRANOLA

Makes 2 servings
Prep time: 25 minutes

Protein Granola

Oil spray (or parchment paper)
½ cup rolled oats
2 tablespoons sliced almonds
3 tablespoons liquid egg whites (or 2 pasture-raised egg whites)
2 teaspoons unfiltered raw honey
2 teaspoons unrefined, cold-pressed coconut oil, melted
½ tablespoon ground flax seed
½ teaspoon ground cinnamon
Dash grated nutmeg
½ scoop vanilla whey or plant protein powder

Apples

1 Honeycrisp apple, cored and sliced very thin
½ teaspoon ground cinnamon
1 teaspoon butter
1 lemon, juiced
1 teaspoon unfiltered raw honey
1 cup full-fat plain or vanilla Skyr or Greek yogurt

1. Preheat the oven to 375°F. Spray a rimmed sheet pan with coconut oil or cover the bottom with parchment paper to prevent sticking.
2. In a medium bowl, combine the remaining protein granola ingredients and toss to coat evenly. Spread the mixture evenly on the prepared sheet pan

and bake for eight minutes. Break up the granola pieces with a spatula or large spoon and bake for eight minutes more, until the mixture starts to crisp.

3. Meanwhile, in a small sauté pan on medium heat, combine the apple, cinnamon, butter, lemon juice, and honey. Cook, stirring continuously, until the apples are softened but not mushy, five to eight minutes.

4. In a small bowl, stir the yogurt until smooth.

5. Assemble the two parfaits. For presentation purposes, a glass cup, martini glass, or clear glass coffee mug would work well. In each glass, layer 1 tablespoon of granola, then a small scoop of yogurt, then the apples and more granola. There's no exact science to this; just continue layering and have fun with it. Serve and enjoy!

PROTEIN PEANUT BUTTER CUPS

Makes 12 servings
Prep time: 30 minutes

Chocolate Shell
  ½ cup dark chocolate chips
  2 tablespoons cacao powder
  2 tablespoons unrefined, cold-pressed coconut oil
  Dash ground cinnamon
  Pinch Himalayan salt

Protein Peanut Butter Filling
  2 tablespoons peanut butter powder
  2 tablespoons unsweetened vanilla almond milk
  ⅓ cup all-natural creamy peanut butter
  1 teaspoon unfiltered raw honey
  stevia powder
  ¼ teaspoon pure vanilla extract
  1 scoop whey or plant protein powder of your choice (chocolate flavor works best)

1. Line a muffin pan with 12 muffin liners.
2. In a medium microwave-safe bowl, combine the chocolate shell ingredients.

(cont.)

Microwave for one minute. Stir until the chocolate chips are fully melted and the mixture is smooth.

3. Spoon about ½ tablespoon of the melted chocolate mixture into each muffin cup, just enough to cover the bottom with a thin layer. After you have filled the cups, carefully tip the pan so the chocolate spreads halfway up the sides of each cup.

4. Freeze the cups for 10 to 15 minutes, until the chocolate hardens.

5. In another medium bowl, combine the peanut butter powder and 1 tablespoon of the almond milk. The peanut butter powder will thicken into a creamy peanut butter consistency. Mix in the natural peanut butter (you may need to microwave the mixture for 30 seconds to soften it for stirring). Add the honey, stevia powder, and vanilla and stir until fully combined. Add the protein powder and the remaining 1 tablespoon of almond milk. Stir to a smooth consistency.

6. Remove the muffin pan from the freezer. Add a 2-teaspoon dollop of the peanut butter mixture to each muffin cup. Smooth it out a bit but leave a little chocolate border around the edges

7. Pour another ½ tablespoon of melted chocolate (microwave to soften, if needed) in each cup, fully encasing the peanut butter mixture.

8. Freeze for about 15 minutes, until the chocolate shell fully hardens. Store in the freezer until ready to eat. Warning: The chocolate melts easily and can get a little messy. Worst-case scenario, you can lick the chocolate off your fingers.

PROTEIN ICE CREAM

Makes 1 bowl
Prep time: 5 minutes (or 45 minutes if you choose to freeze)

1 tablespoon all-natural almond butter
1 scoop chocolate whey or plant protein powder
4 tablespoons dairy milk or unsweetened vanilla plant-based milk of your choice

1. If the almond butter is stiff, place it in a small bowl and melt it for a few seconds in the microwave. Add the protein powder and mix until smooth.
2. Add the milk and slowly whisk the mixture to a pudding-like texture. You can also use a blender. If you're not happy with the consistency, you can always add in a little more milk.
3. If you want, you can eat this right now and call it protein pudding. I prefer to throw it in the freezer for 30 to 45 minutes for an ice cream–like consistency.

PEANUT BUTTER PROTEIN RICE CRISPY TREATS

Makes 16 servings
Prep time: 15 minutes, plus 30 minutes in the freezer

Oil spray
½ cup all-natural creamy peanut butter
¼ cup organic brown rice syrup
¼ cup unfiltered raw honey, more as needed
1 teaspoon pure vanilla extract
2½ cups crispy brown rice cereal
2 scoops vanilla whey or plant protein powder
2 tablespoons unrefined, cold-pressed coconut oil
1 tablespoon cacao (or cocoa) powder
¼ cup dark chocolate chips

1. Grease an 8 x 8-inch Pyrex or metal baking pan with coconut oil spray.
2. In a medium saucepan over medium-low heat, combine the peanut butter, brown rice syrup, honey, and vanilla. Stir until melted and smooth, about two to three minutes. Remove from the heat and stir in the rice cereal and 1 scoop of the protein powder. The mixture should be soft but not runny. If it's too hard to stir with a spoon, mix in a little more honey.
3. Scoop the mixture into the pan and spread it out evenly, pressing it gently to fill the corners.
4. In the same saucepan (it's okay if there's peanut butter residue—there are worse things to worry about in life), combine the coconut oil, cocoa powder, and chocolate chips over medium-high heat. Stir until melted and smooth. Remove from the heat, add the remaining 1 scoop of protein powder, and stir to combine.
5. Top the rice crispies with the protein chocolate topping. Spread it all over to reach the corners.
6. Freeze for 30 minutes, then cut into 16 squares. (Try not to eat the whole thing at once.) It will keep best if refrigerated, but you can store at room temperature. If it becomes crumbly, eat it like granola on top of yogurt or in a bowl with milk. Yum!

FLOURLESS BANANA CHOCOLATE ALMOND MUFFINS

Makes 12 muffins
Prep time: 25 minutes

2 extra-ripe bananas, smashed with a fork (about ¾ cup)
¼ cup full-fat plain Greek yogurt
1 tablespoon all-natural almond butter
1 tablespoon unrefined, cold-pressed coconut oil, melted
⅔ cup liquid egg whites
2 whole pasture-raised eggs
1 teaspoon pure vanilla extract
2 tablespoons unfiltered raw honey
½ cup oat flour (see note)
¼ cup old-fashioned rolled oats
1 teaspoon baking powder
1 teaspoon baking soda
¼ teaspoon Himalayan salt
¼ teaspoon ground cinnamon
¼ cup slivered almonds
2 tablespoons dark chocolate chips

Note: You can purchase oat flour or make your own by grinding oats in a blender or food processor.

1. Preheat the oven to 375°F. Line 12 muffin wells with paper liners.
2. In a large bowl, combine the bananas, yogurt, almond butter, coconut oil, egg whites, eggs, vanilla, and honey and mix well. In another large bowl, combine the oat flour, rolled oats, baking powder, baking soda, salt, cinnamon, almonds, and chocolate chips. Add the dry mixture to the wet mixture and mix until well combined (do not overmix).
3. Using a spoon or an ice cream scoop, divide the batter among the muffin wells, filling them about three-quarters full.
4. Bake for 20 minutes, until the top of the muffins lightly brown. Set aside to cool in the pan, approximately five minutes.
5. Enjoy immediately, store in an airtight container in the fridge for up to a week, or freeze for up to a month.

PB&J ENERGY BALLS

Makes 25 balls
Prep time: 15 minutes

8 Medjool dates, pitted
⅓ cup all-natural creamy peanut butter
2 tablespoons low-sugar jelly or preserves, flavor of your choice
1 teaspoon pure vanilla extract
1 teaspoon unfiltered raw honey
2 scoops whey or plant protein powder (chocolate, vanilla, or unflavored will work)
Dash ground cinnamon
Pinch Himalayan salt
1 tablespoon chia seeds
¼ cup unsalted roasted peanuts
2 tablespoons unsweetened dried cranberries or tart cherries
½ cup rolled oats
Unrefined, cold-pressed coconut oil (optional)

1. In a small bowl, combine the dates and just enough warm water to cover the tops. Let soak for 10 to 15 minutes, until softened.
2. In a food processor, combine the dates, peanut butter, jelly, vanilla, honey, protein powder, cinnamon, and salt. Process until smooth. You may have to stop and use a spatula to scrape down the sides. You're welcome to taste test from the spatula (because you have to make sure it's good so far). Add the chia seeds, peanuts, dried fruit, and oats. Pulse in quick increments to combine while still maintaining some of the texture.
3. Spoon out about a tablespoon of the mixture and roll into a ball about 1 inch thick. Greasing your hands with coconut oil will help you roll the balls easier. Repeat for each ball. Place on parchment paper, seal in a container, and refrigerate.

Chapter 12

THE PLAN THAT NEVER STOPS WORKING

"WHAT HAPPENS WHEN THE plan stops working?"

No matter how much you want to deny it, this question lurks in the back of your mind like Michael Myers. Because even when you think you've killed your dieting demons of the past, they always find a way to come back to life. We're programmed to set expectations based on past experiences.

To answer your question, I'm going to start with a slightly different question: *How do you know when the plan stops working?*

Again, the game we're playing has a different set of rules. It's not, "Oh no, I screwed up and now need to compensate." Instead, it's about creating context of what is normal and what is problematic. When you sense a problem, you overreact, and that sends you on a crash course. If you have a better sense of when to be concerned, it will help you stay calm when you're unsure about the path you're following. And, if you truly fall off track, you'll have plenty of ways to troubleshoot and make your life easier.

YOU WON'T BELIEVE THIS (BUT IT'S TRUE)

A weight-loss plateau can be a very good thing. In fact, if you don't want to regain the weight, a plateau might be a key part of how you prevent the scale from returning to your prior weight.

A key theory in weight loss is known as the set point. We all have that weight that just seems to be "your weight." You might fluctuate a few pounds here or there, but when you think of your weight, a specific number comes to mind that just seems easy to maintain (and not always in the way you want it to). Set points can change over time when you spend long enough at a new weight. This is how you gain weight over time that doesn't happen immediately or easily. Remember, the average person only gains one to three pounds per year after the age of thirty. It's a slow gain rather than big a jump, and this might partially have to do with the set point theory.

Research suggests that some people have higher set points (you stick at a heavier weight) and other people have lower set points (you stick at a lighter weight). The set point is important in the conversation about it being easier to gain weight than lose weight. If you can think of it in the way we are going to discuss, it won't be as frustrating. If you can understand why it happens, you can use plateaus to finally help you lower your set point.

Let's say you go on a diet and lose weight. This doesn't make your brain happy because it's focused on maintaining your current size (your set point). To fight against the drop in weight, your body automatically adjusts. Your metabolism slows down, your hunger increases, and your body desires more caloric foods.

To add to the struggle, as you lose weight, your fat cells shrink. When this happens, they produce less of a hormone (leptin) that tells your brain you don't need food. That's right. As you lose fat, your fat cells stop communicating with your brain, and your brain thinks you need more food. It's messed up—but it makes it easy to understand why so many people either struggle to lose weight or regain what they've lost. However, know that there are ways to work *with* your body so you don't regain the weight.

As I mentioned, people can—and do!—keep the weight off. Those who succeed remove time pressures and emphasize progress and patience. The faster you lose weight, the more aggressively your body is likely to fight back. While fast and slow weight loss can result in long-term success, sometimes it's helpful to take a slower route because of the sanity it provides.

This isn't about figuring out how you can lose weight. Instead, it's thinking about the behaviors you add and change, and how quickly you'll want to abandon them. If you make small changes that lead to one or two pounds of weight loss per month, then you're less likely to revert to old behaviors, and your set point is more likely to change to a lower weight. This approach means losing, pausing and plateauing, and then losing more.

We think that we need to be super strict with our plans, but research paints a different picture. *Diet breaks can be incredibly powerful.* In a study published in the *International Journal of Obesity,* people who cut calories for two weeks—and then took a break for two weeks—lost more weight and body fat than people who stayed on a diet continuously. After six months, those who had a more relaxed approach to eating—while still cutting calories—maintained weight loss of nearly sixteen pounds more than those who followed the strict plan.[1]

While more research is needed, this approach has many potential benefits. For starters, your brain doesn't fight as hard against slower weight loss. And it means your body can adjust to your new body weight and reestablish a lower set point.

For example, let's say your set point is around 180 pounds. You'd love to weigh 160 pounds, but no matter what you do, you seem to hover around 180. The typical approach is to try and lose twenty pounds. This requires lots of big changes, a ton of stress, and a big jump to recalibrate your set point by twenty pounds. After all, you're not just trying to lose twenty pounds; you're trying to make it easier for you to maintain a weight that's twenty pounds lighter than your current weight.

Instead, it's worth making it easier on your body to maintain your new weight. This might mean spending the first one to two months focused on losing the first five pounds. Then, you plateau and allow your body to readjust. Suddenly, 175 is easy to maintain. Then, you drop another five pounds, plateau, and start losing again.

Five pounds is just an example, and you can certainly make bigger jumps. The more you have to lose to be a healthier weight, the bigger the jumps can be, but—at a maximum—one to two pounds per week is the average you should be losing if you want to do it in a healthy and sustainable way. No matter what, it's important to know the following:

- Slower weight loss can be effective when you want to avoid regaining the weight because it doesn't require extreme behaviors that are hard to maintain.
- Think of plateaus as a part of success—allowing you to reset your set point and prevent your brain from fighting against you.

So how do you know when you're off track? You reset your expectations. Being off track is no longer about eating dessert, having carbs, or going a week without weight loss. It's about making sure you're using the tools you've been given in this book. Then, it's a matter of being aware of seeing small steps of progress (like walking more, doing your workouts, and eating protein and fiber) and appreciating that plateaus might be an indication that your body is adjusting and preparing for more success.

As I just mentioned, if you want to lose more than ten pounds, a safe weight loss, on average, is one to two pounds per week—max!

It might be hard because of what you've been taught, but I want you to try to *not* worry about weekly weight loss. Instead, focus more on monthly weight loss. That means, on average, the goal would be about four to five pounds per month. And, as you get closer to your goal, that amount could be cut in half.

Plateaus Are Part of Long-Term Success
ANATOMY OF PROGRESS

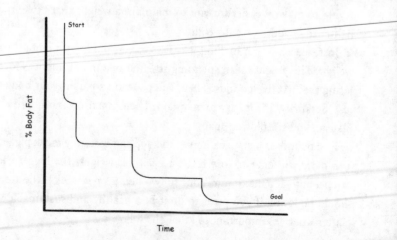

Plateauing is a part of the process that will help you have long-term success and help you get off the rollercoaster of weight loss and regain.

Not to mention, after you lose three to five pounds, it's completely normal—and arguably healthier—to plateau for one to three weeks and not lose much weight at all. Remember, you're creating a new set point, which will make it easier to maintain your new body. It's easy to get frustrated by slower results, but it's time to stop playing checkers and start playing chess.

Would you rather lose twenty pounds in one month and gain it all back—while slowing down your metabolism in the long run? Or would you rather lose four pounds per month over the next six months, enjoy many of the foods you love, recalibrate your set point—and have it feel easier to maintain a weight that's twenty-five pounds lower than you started?

The choice is easy—you just need to be willing to progress slowly and not stress the weeks when you plateau.

WHAT TO DO WHEN YOU'RE STUCK

Don't overreact! That's the first rule of successful body transformation. All too often, when you don't see results quickly (or at all), your impulse is to make a dramatic adjustment. But this will take you on a detour that leaves you far from your goal destination. Sometimes, no adjustment is needed. As we discussed, your body could be adjusting or recalibrating its set point.

That said, if you're truly stalled and you haven't seen any changes for approximately three weeks, then it's time for a quick assessment. Here are the best places to adjust to help jumpstart progress.

Start with Sleep
While the debate about nutrition and exercise gets all the attention, sleep is arguably the most important habit for better health. According to the Centers for Disease Control and Prevention, more than 35 percent of Americans are sleep deprived. And, when you consider that nearly the same percentile is

obese, I'm here to tell you that the statistical similarity is likely more than a coincidence.

Not sleeping enough—less than seven hours of sleep per night—can reduce and undo the benefits of dieting, according to research published in the *Annals of Internal Medicine*.[2]

In the study, dieters were put on different sleep schedules. When their bodies received adequate rest, half the weight they lost was from fat.

However, when they cut back on sleep, the amount of fat lost was cut in half—even on the same diet. What's more, they felt significantly hungrier, were less satisfied after meals, and lacked the energy to exercise. Overall, those on a sleep-deprived diet experienced a 55 percent reduction in fat loss compared to their well-rested counterparts.

Poor Sleep Changes Your Fat Cells

Think about the last time you had a bad night of sleep. How did you feel when you woke up? Exhausted. Dazed. Confused. Maybe even a little grumpy?

It's not just your brain and body that feel that way—your fat cells do, too. When your body is sleep-deprived, it suffers from "metabolic grogginess." The term was coined by University of Chicago researchers who analyzed what happened after just four days of poor sleep[3]—something that commonly happens during a busy week. One late night at work leads to two late nights at home, and next thing you know, you're in sleep debt.

But it's just four nights, so how bad could it be? You might be able to cope just fine. After all, coffee works wonders. But the hormones that control your fat cells don't feel the same way. Within just four days of sleep deprivation, your body's ability to properly use insulin (the master storage hormone) becomes completely disrupted. In fact, the researchers found that insulin sensitivity dropped by more than 30 percent.

Here's why that's bad: When your insulin is functioning well, fat cells remove fatty acids and lipids from your bloodstream and prevent storage. When you become more insulin resistant, fats (lipids) circulate in your blood and pump out more insulin. Eventually, this excess insulin ends up storing fat in all the wrong places, such as tissues like your liver. And this is exactly how you become fat and suffer from diseases like diabetes.

Lack of Rest Makes You Crave Food

Your brain is a central character in how we gain and lose weight. So, it's probably no surprise that a lack of sleep only makes your mind fight against your body even more. Hunger is controlled by two hormones: leptin (which you just learned about) and ghrelin.

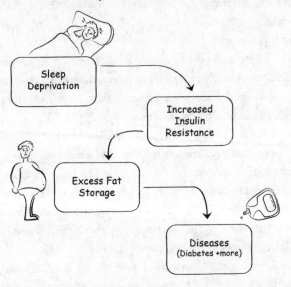

Fix Your Sleep, Transform Your Life

Leptin is a hormone that's produced in your fat cells. The less leptin you produce, the more your stomach feels empty. Leptin is controlled by your fat cells, which is why leptin drops when you lose weight.

The more ghrelin you produce, the more you stimulate hunger while also reducing the number of calories you burn (your metabolism) and increasing the amount of fat you store. In other words, you need to control leptin and ghrelin to successfully lose weight, but sleep deprivation makes that nearly impossible.

There's a mountain of research suggesting that a lack of sleep triggers areas in your brain that increase your need for food by depressing leptin and increasing ghrelin.[4] And while the amount of sleep you "need" can differ, at least one study showed that the domino effect of disruption can begin when you sleep less than seven hours per night.[5]

If that's not enough, scientists discovered exactly how sleep loss creates an internal battle that makes it nearly impossible to lose weight. When you don't sleep enough, your cortisol levels rise. This is the stress hormone frequently associated with fat gain. Cortisol also activates reward centers in your brain that make you want food. At the same time, loss of sleep causes your body to produce more ghrelin. A combination of high ghrelin and cortisol shut down the areas of your brain that leave you feeling satisfied after a meal, meaning you feel hungry all the time—even if you just ate a big meal.

And it gets worse.

Lack of sleep also pushes you in the direction of the foods you know you shouldn't eat. A study published in *Nature Communications* found that just one night of sleep deprivation was enough to impair activity in your frontal lobe, which controls complex decision-making.[6]

Ever had an internal conversation like this? "I really shouldn't have that extra piece of cake . . . then again, one slice won't really hurt, right?"

Turns out, sleep deprivation is a little like being drunk. You just don't have the mental clarity to make good complex decisions, specifically in regard to the foods you eat—or foods you want to avoid. This isn't helped by the fact that when you're overtired, you also have increased activity in the amygdala, the reward region of your brain.

This is why sleep deprivation destroys all diets. Think of the amygdala as mind control—it makes you crave high-calorie foods. Normally you might be able to fight off this desire, but because your insular cortex (another portion of your brain) is weakened due to sleep deprivation, you have trouble fighting the urge and are more likely to indulge in all the wrong foods.

And if all that wasn't enough, research published in *Psychoneuroendocrinology* (say that five times fast) found that sleep deprivation makes you select greater portion sizes of all foods, further increasing the likelihood of weight gain.[7] The bottom line: Not enough sleep means you're always hungry, reaching for bigger portions, and desiring every type of food that you want to limit. If things feel extra hard, start by analyzing your sleep, and make sure you get *at least* seven hours.

The Sleep Boost

Getting more sleep is easier said than done. If you're struggling to get good rest, here are a few recommendations that might help.

EXPOSE YOURSELF TO EARLY SUNLIGHT: Your circadian rhythm helps determine sleep. While most tips focus on what you do before you go to bed, what you do when you wake up might be most important. When you allow light into your eyes early in the morning, it sets a "timer" for your circadian clock that will help you feel sleepier at night. If you can't get five minutes of direct sunlight (think of opening your curtains and looking outside), then just turn on the lights brightly in your home.

DIM THE LIGHTS AT NIGHT: While early sunlight is great, looking at bright lights later at night has the opposite effect. This is one of the reasons late-night screentime can cause a problem. But with phones and other screens, you can easily use a blue light filter. Just make sure you also dim lights when possible, starting about two hours before you sleep.

TIME YOUR SLEEP CYCLE: You sleep in phases. Half a phase is forty-five minutes and a full phase is ninety minutes. Throughout the cycle you go through different depths of sleep—from light to deep. If you wake up in the middle of a phase—even if you've slept a lot—it can make you groggy and tired because you're waking up in deep sleep.

If you want to improve your rest, make sure you sleep in intervals that align with your phases of sleep. I dream of going to bed at 9 pm, but with two young kids, it's not a reality. If I'm in bed by 10 pm, I'll feel more refreshed if I wake up at 5:30 am (7.5 hours of sleep) as opposed to 6 am, simply because I'm working with my sleep cycle rather than against it. When I wake at 5:30, I have timed it for just as my sleep cycle ends so I feel alert and well-rested. Whereas if I got up at 6, I'd have clocked more total hours of sleep, but I likely wouldn't feel like it because I'd be waking up just as I was falling back into a deeper sleep.

TIME YOUR MEALS: You know one of the tools in this book is to create boundaries around your meals. This isn't just to help you eat less; it's also to help you sleep better. If you eat within two hours of sleep, it can reduce your body's natural production of melatonin, a hormone released by your brain to help you sleep. The more melatonin you produce, the easier it is for you to fall asleep faster and stay asleep longer.

TIME YOUR HYDRATION: Good hydration is an essential component of your health, but too much drinking before you sleep can severely disrupt a restful night of sleep, and even cause a disorder known as nocturia. Remove liquids at least one to two hours before you sleep, and while you're at it, try to make smarter drink choices. While a little alcohol might appear to help you sleep faster, it will wake you up sooner and keep you up, as it's a powerful diuretic.

MANAGE YOUR CAFFEINE: A little bit of caffeine will run through your body much longer than you feel it. While your buzz might wear off, caffeine has a half-life of about four to six hours. So, if you have a little pick-me-up cup of coffee at 3 pm, that means *half* of the caffeine could still be in your system at 9 pm. Ever wonder why it can be hard to fall asleep? This is a primary reason for many people.

This has a direct impact on your ability to rest. Researchers found that caffeine six hours before bedtime reduces sleep by more than one hour.[8] Remember how your goal is to sleep at least seven hours? If you're sipping down more coffee later in the afternoon or evening, you're making this an uphill battle. To be on the safe side, cut off caffeine about eight hours before you sleep.

DROP THE TEMPERATURE: Your body sleeps longer in a cooler environment. That's because your body temperature decreases approximately 2°F during the night. If you keep the room too warm, it won't impact how easily you fall asleep, but it will affect how much restorative sleep you get[9] (the slow-wave sleep), decrease your sleep efficiency, and make it more likely that you'll wake up during the night.[10]

MAKE A TO-DO LIST: One of the most underrated ways to help you fall asleep is to remove the thoughts that keep you awake. The simplest way to do so is by writing about them. Researchers at Baylor University found that writing an evening to-do list can improve how quickly you fall asleep.[11] By writing about things on your mind or your plans for the following day, you can decrease distractions, overthinking, and stress, which makes it easier to pass out peacefully.

If you can shift your expectations and prioritize your sleep, you'll immediately find that the journey to better health becomes more enjoyable, less stressful, and easier to navigate. There's less pressure to look for visible success every week, and more time and energy can be dedicated to your habits and the process. The next big shift is putting an end to the competition about what constitutes the "best" diet, which makes it easier than ever to eat in a way that caters to your preferences.

CHAPTER SUMMARY

- Weight loss plateaus are part of the process. When weight loss stalls (if that's your goal), do not freak out or immediately react by cutting more calories. Experiencing two to three weeks where weight loss has stalled is normal. If you stick to your tools and don't overreact, your body will recalibrate and start losing again.
- In general, focus on monthly changes instead of weekly. If you boil it down to weekly outcomes, you'll lose an average of one to two pounds per week. Slow and steady really can win the race.
- If you're struggling, check in on your sleep habits. Sleep deprivation increases hunger, decreases fat burning, and makes all healthy habits much more difficult.

Chapter 13

PUTTING IT ALL TOGETHER

CONFESSION TIME: I REALLY don't like meal plans.

The issue with meal plans is that, on a subconscious level, you think that you must follow the plan to a "T." And, as we've discussed, anything that increases stress and makes you overthink is part of the problem.

At the same time, people love examples. It's because we're all observational learners. In the 1960s, psychologist Albert Bandura explored the nature of social learning theory when he discovered how well children could pick up and mimic behaviors via observation.

The problem? Social learning applies equally to both good and bad. The meal plan that teaches you that you have the freedom to eat can be the same meal plan that makes you feel tethered to particular meals, eaten at certain times, and on specific days.

That's the last thing that should happen.

If you choose to use any part of this meal plan, do so knowing that it's 100 percent adaptable and adjustable to your food preferences, lifestyle, and mealtime preferences.

You have the freedom to eat at the times you prefer, select foods that fit your desires, and adjust in a way that makes you feel your best.

The tools you've been provided are guardrails to help you make better decisions. But within those guardrails, there is plenty of room for you to find your comfort zone.

THE EATING PLAN

These meals are based on the recipes provided, the general takeout guidelines, and restaurant selections from the top fifty list. The number of meals you eat is up to you, but most people tend to do well with three meals spread throughout the day.

I limited the takeout options to a maximum of three times per week, but I suggest starting with one or two times per week. This is merely a recommendation, but it will help you start strong and build better habits.

Change takes time. And the biggest change is the one that will take place between your two ears: believing you're a healthy person.

That won't happen overnight, because old habits die hard, new habits take time to form, and takeout food—while delicious and totally fine—can still be very tempting, especially when you're not at a level when food doesn't cause stress.

So start slow. Walk before you run. And learn to enjoy this new approach. You might have left the old game, but learning a new game—even if it's a better one—still takes time.

I learned to live off takeout five days per week and still lose fat. But it took me time to master that. When I started at that pace without a plan, I gained a lot of weight, lost energy, and struggled.

And, research at the University of Massachusetts found that people who eat more than a third of their meals at restaurants are nearly 70 percent more likely to be obese. If you're eating out just twice per week (with an average of twenty-one meals per week—three meals per day, seven days per week), then 90 percent of your meals are of the homemade variety. That's great.

Even at three takeout orders per week, you're still far ahead of the 67 percent cut-off, meaning you're statistically more likely to be healthy—while having flexibility—which is a great place to be.

If you need a reminder to keep you on track, I like to tell people to think of the three Ps: patience, progression, and personalization:

- Be patient as you explore your newfound freedom.
- Progress (and expand your comfort zone) when things feel easy, you feel better, and you're seeing the results you want.
- Personalize it so the plan fits your lifestyle best.

Just because you can eat takeout doesn't mean you have to. When I'm not traveling, I have takeout twice per week: Fridays for pizza night and Saturday for date night. I can eat out more often without worry, but two times per week is what works best for me and my family.

Like everything else in this book, you don't need to figure it out right away—and there's no deadline for having it all together, if you ever do!

We live in a world where everyone acts like they always have their shit together, and that pressure is both a false reality and an unnecessary stress.

Remember that something is better than nothing. You do the best you can to use the tools, even if it's just maintaining eating boundaries and slowing down the pace of your meal. Avoid those zero percent weeks, and you'll be as perfect as you ever need to be.

And, if you have a "zero" week, just know it happens to everyone. Laugh it off. Order some good takeout and get back at it.

If you lose your way, that's what this meal plan is really for. It's another support system to remind you that you've got this.

Sound good? Let's eat.

MEAL SUPPORT

Even with the best plan, it's easy to wonder if something is off. Whenever doubt creeps in your mind, here are several ways to check in with your progress and your process to make sure you're doing the things that will make your life easier.

If you're in a true plateau, it's possible that you're not using some of the tools, or you might be unknowingly doing things that lead to overeating. Here are a few subtle decisions that can throw you off course.

How often are you eating takeout?

As you know, I think cooking more meals at home and embracing takeout is part of a sustainable approach that supports long-term success. However, you can have too much of a good thing. If you're finding that you're struggling to achieve your goals, check how often you're eating takeout. The sweet spot is one to three times per week. If you're eating out more often, cut it back for a couple of weeks and see what happens.

Are you eating takeout or going to restaurants?

No offense to restaurants, but their environment is littered with landmines. If you recall the lessons from Stephan Guyenet, controlling your environment to reduce temptation makes it much easier to control your eating. Even if you're full or not craving foods, environmental signals can flip on the "eat more food" switch and lead to overeating.

When in doubt it's better to be in an environment where it's harder to easily reward yourself with food. Stick to takeout when possible and leave trips to restaurants for special occasions.

Are you a big snacker?

Many years ago, it was suggested that small, frequent meals were the ideal way to eat for fat loss. It was based on the idea that eating more often would boost your metabolism. But there was just one small problem: The theory never held up when tested.

Fast forward many years, and researchers have tirelessly tried to prove that eating more often helps with fat loss. Try as they may, as of this writing, not a single study has found a difference in calories burned as you increase meal frequency (assuming calories and macronutrients are equal). In other words, if you eat the same amount and types of food and split them up into many or fewer meals, it has no impact on your metabolism. Researchers have compared anywhere from one meal to seven meals within a twenty-four-hour period and found no difference in the total number of calories you burn in a day.[1]

On the surface, this means you should find the number of meals that work for you. But there's an exception to the rule. The research depends on snacking not leading to more eating. And sometimes, a little snack can open the floodgates to more eating.

Even if you have the best intentions, research suggests that eating a little less often might make it easier to eat less,[2] simply because you're not around food as often. Not to mention, because you won't be counting calories, you'll want to be aware of blind spots. And one of the biggest blind spots is assessing food intake. Research has found that people underestimate their food intake by an average of 47 percent.[3] So the more often you eat, the more likely you are to underestimate how much you're eating, which is where frustration and overeating can happen. With the tools you've been provided, you're more likely to get full and not overeat. But each additional meal is an opportunity to eat more than you want. If you're a big snacker and you're struggling, try cutting back the snacks for a week or two and see what happens.

Find Your Trouble Spot

Everyone has one meal that's most difficult. When I surveyed a group of five hundred people who tested the plan in this book, the group complained equally about the difficulties of breakfast, lunch, and dinner. And that should come as no surprise. Your lifestyle dictates the meals that create the most friction.

The key to dealing with your trouble meal is making the obstacle the way. Instead of just hoping the one trouble meal will improve, replace it completely. Now, I'm not suggesting skipping the meal. However, finding an "easy button" is a way to troubleshoot something that creates stress or is making it harder for you to accomplish your goals.

The "easy buttons" are the four Ss: soup, salad, sandwich, or smoothie. Simply take the meal you struggle with most and substitute it with one of the four Ss. The key is making sure you prep these meals the right way. Here is your blueprint.

Soups

Look for soups that are less than 300 calories, contain at least 5 grams of fiber, and, ideally, have more than 15 grams of protein. You'll see options in the recipes section.

Sandwiches

They have a bad reputation, but sandwiches can be a staple of a healthy diet. Here's how to build the ultimate healthy sandwich.

Build Your Base

Bread, Tortilla or Wrap

Ideally, select a high-fiber bread. Look for an option with at least 4 grams of fiber in a single serving. Does it always need to be high-fiber? No. Don't stress if you grab a few slices of white bread every now and then. If you go high-fiber about 80 percent of the time, consider that 100 percent perfection.

Add a High-Fiber Veggie or Fruit

Black beans, lentils, sprouts, carrots, kale or spinach, sliced pear, banana

Add Protein

Chicken, turkey, lean beef, fish, tempeh, tofu, egg

Add a Healthy Fat

Avocado, olive or avocado oil, flaxseed, sunflower seed, chia seeds

Add Flavor

Hot sauce, Greek yogurt, avocado mayo, salt and pepper, balsamic

Salad

No surprise, but salads are a quick fix when you need a meal that is super filling. Salads can check all the boxes—high in protein and fiber, easy to eat slowly, and typically low in ultra-processed foods. Plus, you can make them quickly and without breaking the bank. The downfall of most salads are the dressings. To keep that in check, think about adding just one spoonful of a dressing. Or, if you're adding olive oil, simply fill the cap, pour it over your salad, and mix.

Smoothie

This is all about nutrient density. You can pack a lot of satisfaction into one drink, and all you need to know is how to use a blender.

- Place 1 or 2 handfuls of ice in a blender.
- Add 8 ounces of water, milk, or a milk substitute: Dairy milk, coconut milk, almond milk, oat milk, pea milk . . . so many options

- Add 1 to 2 servings of protein: Try whey protein powder, plant protein powder, Greek yogurt, cottage cheese, or soft tofu
- Add 2 servings of vegetables: Grab two big handfuls of spinach, kale, or cauliflower, or a serving of greens powder. You can get creative, but these mix best and have minimal impact on flavor.
- 1 serving natural sweetness: Banana, berries, or dates
- 1 spoonful fat: Avocado, nut butter, chia seeds, flax seeds (optional)

The supplement industry is a messy and hard to trust. I would know because I played in it for several years when I was a founding member and chief nutrition officer of Ladder. Most supplements are a complete waste of money, but there are a few that I think are helpful. My favorite "supplement" is protein powder.

There's nothing special about protein powder compared to whole food sources of protein. But, as you know, protein is a key foundation of a healthy eating plan. And, most diets tend to be low in high-quality proteins. That's why I like having protein shakes. The good ones are a clean source of protein, and they maximize convenience (only takes a few minutes to make). Plus, research shows that supplementing with a meal replacement (like a protein powder) is an effective way to be more in control of your diet (and support weight loss, if that's your goal). If you're looking for a good protein powder, make sure you choose a brand that has a third-party certification like NSF, Informed Sport, or BSCG. This ensures the quality, purity, and safety of the product. I recommend Vitalura Protein, which was created by a good friend (Anna Victoria) who deeply cares about creating supplements the right way. Tastes great, no crap, and gives your body a healthy dose of protein. If you're looking for a meal replacement with fiber-loaded carbs, protein, and healthy fat, then there is no better option than Meal One by Kreatures of Habit.

WEEK 1

Monday
Breakfast: Creamy Strawberry Smoothie
Lunch: Protein High-Protein Grilled Cheese
Takeout Dinner: 8-piece cut roll + 6 pieces assorted sashimi

Tuesday
Breakfast: Omelet Muffins
Lunch: Mediterranean Rotisserie Pita
Dinner: Steak Stir-Fry

Wednesday
Takeout Breakfast: Egg White Bites (Starbucks)
Lunch: Steak Sandwich
Dinner: Slow-Cooker High-Protein Sweet Potato Chili

Thursday
Breakfast: Mocha Protein Shake
Lunch: Leftover chili
Dinner: Naked Chicken Tenders + Apple and Bacon-Roasted Brussels Sprouts

Friday
Breakfast: Peanut Butter–Banana Overnight Oats
Lunch: Honey Mustard Chicken BLT Wrap
Takeout Dinner/Bliss Meal: Pizza night

Saturday
Breakfast: Bacon and Date Protein Pancakes
Lunch: Feta and Chickpea Quinoa Salad
Dinner: Buffalo Chicken Quesadilla

Sunday
Breakfast: Veggie Egg Sandwich
Lunch: Avocado Tuna Salad
Dinner: Peanut Pad Thai and Shrimp

WEEK 2

Monday
Breakfast: Mocha Protein Shake
Lunch: Buffalo Chicken Quesadilla (leftovers from Saturday)
Dinner: Caprese Bison Burgers

Tuesday
Takeout Breakfast: Veggie Egg White Flatbread (Dunkin')
Lunch: Avocado Tuna Salad (leftovers from Sunday)
Dinner: Slow-Cooker High-Protein Sweet Potato Chili

Wednesday
Breakfast: Scrambled eggs (3 eggs) + High-fiber toast
Lunch: Peanut Pad Thai and Shrimp
Dinner: Taco Salad

Thursday
Breakfast: Oatmeal + 1 scoop of protein powder
Lunch: Slow-Cooker High-Protein Sweet Potato Chili (leftovers from Tuesday)
Dinner: Protein Nachos

Friday
Breakfast: Peaches and Greens Smoothie Bowl
Takeout Lunch: Turkey Tom (Jimmy John's)
Dinner: Shrimp Tacos

Saturday
Breakfast: Chai Protein Shake with Maca Powder
Lunch: Shrimp wrap (with leftover shrimp from last night's dinner)
Dinner: Sweet Potato Mac-n-Cheese with Bacon

Sunday
Breakfast: Cinnamon Raisin French Toast Sticks
Lunch: Chicken Noodle Soup
Takeout Dinner: Pizza night

WEEK 3

Monday
Breakfast: Peanut Butter–Banana Overnight Oats
Lunch: Chicken Noodle Soup
Dinner: Fish Foil Packets

Tuesday
Breakfast: Oatmeal + 1 scoop of protein powder
Lunch: Sweet Potato Mac-n-Cheese with Bacon (leftovers)
Dinner: Naked Tenders + Broccoli salad

Wednesday
Breakfast: Chai Protein Shake with Maca Powder
Takeout Lunch: California Dreaming Sub (Jersey Mike's)
Dinner: Baked Salmon and Veggies

Thursday
Breakfast: Oatmeal + 1 scoop of protein powder
Lunch: Double Avocado Salad with Chicken (El Pollo Loco)
Dinner: Chicken Burritos

Friday
Breakfast: Peaches and Greens Smoothie Bowl
Lunch: Buffalo Chicken Quesadilla (with leftover chicken from last night's dinner)
Dinner: Caprese Bison Burgers

Saturday
Takeout Breakfast: Eggs + Turkey Bacon + Sourdough Toast (IHOP)
Lunch: Mediterranean Rotisserie Pita
Dinner: Taco Salad

Sunday
Breakfast: Creamy Strawberry Smoothie
Lunch: Avocado Tuna Salad
Dinner: Steak Stir-Fry

WEEK 4

Monday
Breakfast: Oatmeal + 1 scoop of protein powder
Lunch: Steak Sandwich (with leftover steak from Sunday)
Takeout Dinner: Chicken Fajitas (Chili's)

Tuesday
Breakfast: Mocha Protein Shake
Lunch: Avocado Tuna Salad (leftovers from Sunday)
Dinner: Sweet Potato Mac-n-Cheese with Bacon

Wednesday
Breakfast: Peanut Butter–Banana Overnight Oats
Lunch: Sweet Potato Mac-n-Cheese with Bacon (leftovers)
Dinner: Peanut Pad Thai and Shrimp

Thursday
Breakfast: Oatmeal + 1 scoop of protein powder
Lunch: Shrimp wrap (leftover shrimp from last night's dinner)
Dinner: Caprese Bison Burgers

Friday
Breakfast: Chocolate-Banana–Peanut Butter Protein Smoothie
Takeout Lunch: Grilled Nuggets (Chick-fil-A)
Dinner: Baked Fish and Veggies

Saturday
Breakfast: Veggie Egg Sandwich
Lunch: Chicken Noodle Soup
Takeout Dinner: Steak Medallions (The Cheesecake Factory)

Sunday
Breakfast: Bacon and Date Protein Pancakes
Lunch: High-Protein Grilled Cheese
Dinner: Chicken Tacos

WEEK 5

Monday
Breakfast: Peanut Butter–Banana Overnight Oats
Lunch: Honey Mustard Chicken BLT Wrap (using leftover chicken from Sunday night)
Dinner: Fish Foil Packets

Tuesday
Breakfast: Oatmeal + 1 scoop of protein powder
Lunch: Chicken Noodle Soup (leftovers from Saturday)
Dinner: Protein Nachos

Wednesday
Takeout Breakfast: Veggie Egg White Flatbread (Dunkin')
Lunch: Mediterranean Rotisserie Pita
Dinner: Chicken Burritos

Thursday
Breakfast: Peaches and Greens Smoothie Bowl
Lunch: Buffalo Chicken Quesadilla (with leftover chicken from last night's dinner)
Dinner: Peanut Pad Thai and Shrimp

Friday
Breakfast: Oatmeal + 1 scoop of protein powder
Lunch: Shrimp Wrap (with leftover shrimp from last night's pad Thai)
Takeout Dinner: Pizza night

Saturday
Breakfast: Cinnamon Raisin French Toast Sticks
Takeout Lunch: Red's Chili Chili (Red Robin)
Dinner: Steak Stir-Fry

Sunday
Breakfast: Cracker Barrel Good Morning Breakfast
Lunch: Chocolate Peanut Butter–Banana Smoothie
Dinner: Slow-Cooker High-Protein Sweet Potato Chili

WEEK 6

Monday
Breakfast: Chai Protein Shake with Maca Powder
Lunch: Steak Sandwich (leftover steak from Saturday)
Dinner: Taco Salad

Tuesday
Breakfast: Oatmeal + 1 scoop of protein powder
Lunch: Slow-Cooker High-Protein Sweet Potato Chili (leftovers from Sunday)
Dinner: Fish Foil Packets

Wednesday
Breakfast: Oatmeal + 1 scoop of protein powder
Takeout Lunch: Grilled Tenders + Wedges (Buffalo Wild Wings)
Dinner: Sweet Potato Mac-n-Cheese with Bacon

Thursday
Takeout Breakfast: Egg White Bites (Starbucks)
Lunch: Sweet Potato Mac-n-Cheese with Bacon (leftovers from Wednesday)
Dinner: Caprese Bison Burger

Friday
Breakfast: Mocha Protein Shake
Lunch: Mediterranean Rotisserie Pita
Takeout Dinner: 6-ounce Filet (Outback)

Saturday
Breakfast: Peanut Butter–Banana Overnight Oats
Lunch: Turkey Tacos
Dinner: Baked Fish and Veggies

Sunday
Breakfast: Bacon and Date Protein Pancakes
Lunch: High-Protein Grilled Cheese
Takeout Dinner: Fajitas (Chili's)

PART 4

YOU CAN'T SCREW UP THIS WORKOUT PLAN

Chapter 14

MOVEMENT MEDICINE: THE 6-WEEK PLAN

GONE ARE THE DAYS when you need to spend sixty to ninety minutes per day in the gym. If you have the time, you can train that way. But it's just not necessary for great results, and there are significant downsides for the average person.

Success is not dependent on the amount of time you spend exercising. It's more about consistency and intensity. Start your workout; keep it simple, focused, and hard; and then get out. Extreme workouts that go on . . . and on . . . and on . . . seemingly help you burn a lot of calories. But there are a few issues.

The more calories you burn from exercise, the more your metabolism downshifts to burn fewer calories when at rest.[1] Again, another seemingly frustrating aspect of the human body, but the entire approach of what you've learned in this book will help keep you headed in the right direction. Weight loss and gain is a relatively simple equation of calories in versus calories out. The complicated part is how calories in and calories out are calculated. Remember, your metabolism has three primary components: your BMR (basal metabolic rate, or the calories you burn just living and breathing), the calories you burn from your diet, and the calories you burn from exercise. The total amount is called your total daily energy expenditure, or TDEE.

And the latest research suggests that you can increase your TDEE, but only up to a point. The more calories you burn during exercise, the more your body appears to slow down your BMR to burn fewer total calories. And the more you exercise, the more your body starts to become efficient and burn fewer calories both during exercise and from your BMR. For example, scientists examined marathon runners during a six-week period. At the start of the study, the runners would burn approximately 6,200 calories per day. At the end of the study, even though they were running the same distances, the runners were only burning 4,900 calories per day.[2] They were still burning calories, but their body adjusted—likely from their BMR. In other words, your body tries to limit the "calories out" side of the equation.

Researchers believe that your body has a threshold that won't allow you to burn significantly more calories than you can replenish. Scientists believe this number is approximately two and a half times your basal metabolic rate. When you approach that number, the calories you burn from exercise start to decrease and so does your resting metabolic rate. This isn't just an exercise consideration; it's about survival. Scientists found the same thing with the hunter-gatherer Hadza. Even though they walk miles and miles per day, their daily metabolism adjusts to make sure their calorie burn doesn't far surpass their calorie intake.

You might be thinking, "So, exercise doesn't work?" Not exactly. There are hundreds of studies that show **exercise is one of the best things you can do for your health, including improving fat loss,** allowing you to eat more carbs, maintaining your youthfulness, immune support, injury prevention, and brain health. Not to mention, the same researchers who found that your BMR can decrease the more you exercise also found that exercise is one of the best ways to help you maintain weight loss. This can't be understated. You've read a lot about how common it is to *regain* weight. One of the best ways to prevent that outcome is by moving your body. Exercise boosts your mood, helps you sleep better, prevents you from getting sick, and gives your body what it needs to fight against diseases like diabetes and heart disease. When you move, your body wins.

The lesson? Working out is important, essential, and good for your body. But you really can't out-exercise a bad diet. If you simply train for endless hours and expect the calories to burn up, your body will create limits and you'll be frustrated.

There's a positive side to this, as you'll see in a moment. It means you don't need to exercise for hours and hours every day. It's harder to consistently find time for a sixty-minute workout every day of the week than something much shorter and only a few times per week.

Another reason to be mindful of the duration of your workouts is the impact they have on your hunger. As we've discussed, so much about feeling in control of eating is learning to control and manage hunger through satisfaction. Long workouts are more likely to increase hunger and trigger stress hormones, which can make it harder to stick to your plan.

Because consistency is king, this plan is designed to outsmart the common reasons most people can't stick to a workout. It's usually some combination of time, confidence, and comfort. And, once again, you'll need to expand your comfort zone. If you're not regularly exercising, you're doing harm to your body. But that doesn't mean you need to spend hours training every day. Instead, you need to play a new game that challenges your body in a way you can sustain.

That said, a great workout plan has a little less flexibility than your diet. Exercise requires a little more structure than food because, for most people, building an exercise habit is different than an eating habit. You're going to eat every day, and you don't need to be reminded to do so. But most people struggle to exercise consistently. So having a structure that creates more consistency—while still providing flexibility—will help you move more often and experience all the benefits that will help you achieve your health goals.

Also, your body reacts to exercise in a specific way. Just as hunger increases as you lose weight and you need ways to outsmart your brain and body, your muscles also adapt once they are challenged. If you do the same thing every day, your body stops adapting and you don't see the same benefits. A good exercise plan is built on a principle of "progressive overload." This simply means that as time goes on, you make slight adjustments so that your body keeps adapting and improving. You don't need to change the exercises at each workout or "confuse" your muscles. You just need to make slight changes that make the workouts a little bit harder. Your body will rise to the challenge, become stronger, and adapt in ways that make you healthier and more resilient.

There's a reason you've invested a lot of sweat in other programs without seeing your body change. You need to make your metabolism work for you by knowing how to take advantage of the three primary components. We have the food part covered. Now it's time to adjust for the other aspects (calories burned from exercise and movement and your basal metabolic rate, which is influenced by lean muscle). When you eliminate the inefficiencies and unnecessary movements and focus on strength and general movement (even something as simple as walking), and also work with your diet to change how your body processes food, you'll reshape the way you look in a fraction of the time.

This six-week exercise program is built around shorter workouts, fewer exercises, and movements that will challenge your muscles more effectively by combining strength with metabolic conditioning. But if done consistently, this can serve as so much more than just a six-week fitness reset. It's a guide that you can use for months because as you become stronger, you can restart the program with your added strength and cardiovascular health. Remember, it's about progressive overload. If at the beginning of the program you could lift only 10 pounds and by the end you can lift 20, when you restart the program again with your newfound strength, it will be a new challenge that will result in your body continuing to change and improve. With exercise, the secret really is about consistency and progression. It doesn't have to be fancy, complicated, or overly long, but it does have to be done repeatedly.

Each workout consists of a primary strength movement to help you build muscle and a metabolic circuit (a few exercises paired together with limited rest), which help you burn more calories, improve your heart health, and increase your mobility, so you suffer from fewer aches and pains. Every workout is less than thirty minutes, and you'll never need to exercise more than three to four times per week.

You'll see two different versions of the plan: a six-week plan that requires minimal equipment (think dumbbells, barbell, and bands) and a four-week bodyweight version (bands are the only equipment you need). This is done intentionally. The plans are designed to help you make progress, regardless of your level of expertise. That said, the equipment versions will be a little harder because of the additional weight. So, if you're new to working out or haven't exercised in a while, the bodyweight version might be a great place to start. And, after four weeks on the bodyweight plan, I recommend you graduate to the equipment plan, as your body will be ready for the additional weight.

But note that the bodyweight plan isn't just for beginners. Everything about this book is designed for real life, and in real life, some days or weeks you don't have time to go to the gym, and you might want to make sure you complete your workouts. When those days happen, feel free to substitute in a bodyweight workout or shift to the bodyweight plan. The plans include similar movements and are designed the same way. All of the weeks align, and if you're in week four or beyond of the equipment program, just follow the week four workouts from the bodyweight version. That way, you can substitute a bodyweight plan if you don't have time to go to the gym, and still stay on your plan. To help you with the workouts, you can find detailed exercise descriptions and tips starting on page 245.

To make the most of these workouts, I highly recommend setting a weekly schedule. As I mentioned, you only need to exercise three or four days per week. Ideally, you'll take a day off after each workout. Just as you create an eating schedule (Tool #1: setting eating boundaries), committing to exercise days makes it easier to hold yourself accountable. The key is being as specific as possible.

Remember, you only need thirty minutes (or less) for these workouts. So, pick your days, schedule a time (as if it were an appointment or meeting), set a reminder in your calendar, and put it on repeat each week. As much as possible, it helps to have a set day and time for your exercise. All you need is consistency and effort to make dramatic results, which is why these workouts are built around a realistic time commitment for your schedule, while they still ensure you're giving your body what it needs. When you make movement part of your routine, it becomes automatic, and that's when you'll finally have results to show for your hard work.

You can schedule the workouts as you want, but—ideally—you won't train on back-to-back days. And, if you can, try to have a day of rest between workouts three and four. Otherwise, simply follow the approach for each day.

One other thing. I'm a big believer in the benefits of walking. The reason is simple. All movement contributes to about 20 to 30 percent of your metabolism, broken up into two components—EAT and NEAT. These are simple acronyms for complicated terms (exercise activity thermogenesis and non-exercise activity thermogenesis). EAT consists of traditional exercise, including walking, whereas NEAT focuses on things like fidgeting, cleaning around your house, and other movement that is not technically activity and therefore often overlooked as exercise. As it turns out, both can have a significant impact on your exercise metabolism. So, instead of feeling like you need to go to the gym, just going on a walk and having nervous energy and a need to move (even if it's just tapping your foot repeatedly while sitting) can have many benefits.

To improve your exercise-based movement, set a goal for 8,000 steps per day—at a minimum, 5,000 steps every day. This can be tough for me and others who have a desk job, so I set two timers every day to remind me to go for short ten-minute walks. Approximately twenty minutes a day of walking will usually get you to 5K. And, with the rest of your daily life movement, it will help make it easier to hit those 8,000 steps.

ISN'T THE RULE 10,000 STEPS?

Do you ever wonder where some of our fitness "best practices" come from? We repeat some things so often we assume they're probably correct. But not all of our commonly accepted fitness axioms have a basis in science. Enter the idea of walking 10,000 steps a day for health. That number started as a marketing strategy that wasn't based on any science.

"In 1965, a Japanese company was selling pedometers, and they gave it a name that, in Japanese, means 'the 10,000-step meter.'" says I-Min Lee, a professor of epidemiology at Harvard University's T.H. Chan School of Public Health. The 10,000 steps goal was basically created to sell more 1960's Fitbits.

So, should you be walking 10,000 steps per day? In general, it's a good goal that has many benefits. But it might not be the *minimum* you need to hit in order to experience benefits.

To examine how many steps you need, Professor Lee led a study that examined step totals and mortality rates in elderly women. Her team found that women who walked more than 4,400 steps per day improved their mortality. Those mortality rates continued to lower before leveling out around 7,500 steps a day.

So, you're likely to get significant health benefits from as little as 5,000 steps a day and hit your stride (pun intended) around 8,000 steps per day. That's not to say that if you walk more you might not see benefits. Rather, it's to set a goal you can realistically achieve knowing it will do your body good.

THE WORKOUTS

Every workout is just twenty to thirty minutes. If you go to a gym, you can spend the additional time getting in extra movement by doing something low intensity, such as walking on a treadmill, spinning, rowing, or playing a sport like swimming or basketball.

Intensity is the main focus of the workouts. This is about maximizing every minute to get the most out of your workouts and your metabolism, without spending more time that won't deliver more results. I want you to push each set hard, but at a weight you feel in complete control of every rep. If that means just using your bodyweight, then use your bodyweight.

Week 1 Workouts

For the first week, your goal is to perform three to four workouts. This applies to both the weight and bodyweight version of the plan. There are a total of four workouts per week, but—as you'll see—perfection is never the goal. It's consistency. If you can only get in three workouts this week, that's still a win.

Week 1: Weight/Equipment Workout

Day 1: Lower Body

WARM-UP

Hip raise: 2 sets x 12 reps
Bodyweight lunge: 2 sets x 12 reps/leg
Dead bug: 2 sets x 8 reps/side

STRENGTH

Perform two to three warm-up sets with a lighter weight. Then, complete three to four sets of the exercise below. Warm-up sets of an exercise help you prepare for the movement by doing them with lighter weight. Let's say you want to use 20 pounds for an exercise. Do one warm-up set with 5 pounds, then a second warm-up set with 10 pounds, and then "working" (non-warm-up) sets with 20 pounds.

Goblet squat: 5 to 6 reps (use a weight you can perform for 7 to 8 reps)

METABOLIC CIRCUIT

Set a timer for eight minutes. Complete as many rounds of this three-exercise circuit as possible, resting as little as needed.

Dumbbell reverse lunge (alternating): 8 reps/leg
Plank row: 12 reps/arm
Dumbbell step-up (bodyweight okay): 15 reps

Day 2: Upper Body

WARM-UP

Kneeling reach through to rotation: 2 sets x 6 reps/side
Inchworm: 2 sets x 8 reps
Band pull-apart: 2 sets x 10 reps

STRENGTH

Perform two to three warm-up sets with a lighter weight. Then, complete three to four sets of the exercise below.

Dumbbell single-arm row: 5 to 6 reps/arm (use a weight you can perform for 7 to 8 reps)

METABOLIC CIRCUIT
Set a timer for eight minutes. Complete as many rounds of this three-exercise circuit as possible, resting as little as needed.

Dumbbell single-arm overhead press: 8 reps
Dumbbell chest-supported row: 12 reps
Push-up: 10 to 20 reps (on a bench or bar or from your knees)

Day 3: Total Body

WARM-UP
Set a timer for three minutes and do 5 reps each of:

Bodyweight squats
Jumping jacks
Push-up
Bodyweight lunge
Inchworm

Try to cycle through two to three times and let the fun begin.

METABOLIC CIRCUIT
Do two warm-up sets of only 3 reps each with a light weight. Then, perform five rounds of this four-exercise complex. Start with a weight you can sustain for 8 to 12 reps.

Dumbbell single-arm overhead press: 6 reps
Dumbbell Romanian deadlift: 6 reps
Dumbbell bent-over row: 6 reps
Dumbbell squat: 6 reps

Day 4: Total Body

WARM-UP

Perform 5 reps on each side of this one incredible move. It might take a few reps to get the hang of it, but it'll loosen up your entire body and have you ready to train.

World's greatest stretch: 5 rounds per side

METABOLIC CIRCUIT

Set a timer for twenty-five minutes. Do the first exercise for twenty seconds, then rest for forty seconds. Cycle through each exercise, starting at the beginning when you finish, until time is up.

Dumbbell reverse lunge (alternating)
Push-up
Dumbbell squat
Hollow body hold
Bodyweight single-leg Romanian deadlift (left leg)
Dumbbell bent-over row
Bodyweight single-leg Romanian deadlift (right leg)
Dumbbell squat + overhead press

Week 1: Bodyweight Workout

Day 1: Lower Body

WARM-UP

Hip raise: 2 sets x 12 reps
Bodyweight lunge: 2 sets x 12 reps/leg
Dead bug: 2 sets x 8 reps/side

STRENGTH

Perform two to three warm-up sets of 5 to 6 reps of the exercise below (squats). Then, complete three to four sets of the exercise below. Rest for about two minutes between sets.

Bodyweight squat: 10 to 20 reps with a four-second hold at the bottom
Perform a bodyweight squat. As you reach the bottom of the movement, stay in the squat position for four seconds (also called a four-second isometric hold), then stand back up. The goal minimum is 10 reps. The maximum is 20. Do what works for your fitness level.

METABOLIC CIRCUIT
Set a timer for eight minutes. Complete as many rounds of this three-exercise circuit as possible, resting as little as needed.

Bodyweight reverse lunge (alternating): 8 reps/leg
Plank (if you can, do alternating shoulder taps): 20 seconds
Step-up: 15 reps

Day 2: Upper Body

WARM UP
Kneeling reach through to rotation: 2 sets x 6 reps/side
Inchworm: 2 sets x 8 reps
T-Superman: 2 sets x 6 reps/side

STRENGTH
Perform two to three warm-up sets of 5 to 6 reps with a light weight. Then, complete three to four sets of the exercise below.

Bodyweight row *or* T-superman: 10 to 15 reps + hold one-second at the top of the movement (squeezing shoulder blades together)

METABOLIC CIRCUIT
Set a timer for eight minutes. Complete as many rounds of this three-exercise circuit as possible, resting as little as needed.

Band pull-apart: 10 to 15 reps
Band single-arm row: 10 to 20 reps
Push-up: 10 to 20 reps (can do on a bench or bar or from your knees)

Day 3: Total Body

WARM-UP

Set a timer for three minutes and do 10 reps each of:

Bodyweight squat
Jumping jacks
Push-up
Lunge
Inchworm

Try to cycle through two to three times and let the fun begin.

METABOLIC CIRCUIT

First, do two warm-up sets of only 3 reps each. Then perform five rounds of
this four-exercise complex.

Band overhead press: 10 reps
Bodyweight single-leg Romanian deadlift: 8 reps/leg
Band seated row: 10 to 20 reps
Bodyweight squat: 10 to 20 reps

Day 4: Total Body

WARM-UP

Perform 5 reps on each side of this one incredible move. It might take a few
reps to get the hang of it, but it'll loosen up your entire body and have you
ready to train.

World's greatest stretch: 5 rounds per side

METABOLIC CIRCUIT

Set a timer for twenty-five minutes. Do the first exercise for twenty seconds,
then rest for forty seconds. Cycle through each exercise, starting at the
beginning when you finish the last one, until time is up.

Bodyweight lunge (alternating)
Push-up
Bodyweight squat
Hollow body hold
Bodyweight single-leg Romanian deadlift (left leg)
Mountain climbers
Bodyweight single-leg Romanian deadlift (right leg)
Superman

Week 2 Workouts

Once again week, the goal is to complete three to four workouts. There are a total of four workouts here, but—remember—perfection is never the goal. It's consistency. If you can get in only three workouts this week, that's still a win. And then, you can start next week with the fourth workout in the series.

You can schedule the workouts as you want, but—ideally—don't train on back-to-back days. That said, it's easier to do day one and day two back-to-back. Whereas, if you can, try to have a day of rest between workout three and workout four.

Otherwise, simply follow the approach for each day.

This week, try to get a minimum of 6,000 steps every day, with a stretch goal of 8,000 steps.

Just like week one, every workout is just twenty to thirty minutes. If you go to a gym, you can spend the additional time getting in extra movement by doing something low intensity, such as walking on a treadmill, spinning, rowing, or a sport like swimming or basketball.

Remember: Intensity is the name of the game. Shorter workouts allow you to push harder because you won't be training for very long. I want you to push each set hard, but at a weight you feel in complete control of every rep. If that means just using your bodyweight, then use your bodyweight.

Week 2: Weight/Equipment Workout

Day 1: Lower Body

WARM-UP
Hip raise: 2 sets x 12 reps
Bodyweight lunge: 2 sets x 12 reps/leg
Dead bug: 2 sets x 10 reps/side

STRENGTH
Perform two to three warm-up sets of both exercises, using a lighter weight. Then, do one exercise, rest thirty seconds, and then do the next exercise. Complete two rounds total.

Goblet squat: 7 to 8 reps (use a weight you can handle for 10 to 12 reps) (rest thirty seconds)
Dumbbell Romanian deadlift: 7 to 8 reps (use a weight you can handle for 10 to 12 reps) (rest two minutes and then repeat once more)

METABOLIC CIRCUIT
Set a timer for eight minutes. Complete as many rounds of this three-exercise circuit as possible, resting as little as needed.

Dumbbell reverse lunge (alternating): 8 reps/leg
Plank row: 12 reps/arm
Dumbbell step-up (bodyweight okay): 15 reps

Day 2: Upper Body

WARM-UP
Kneeling reach through to rotation: 2 sets x 6 reps/side
Inchworm: 2 sets x 8 reps
Band pull-apart: 2 sets x 10 reps

STRENGTH
Perform two to three warm-up sets. Then, complete two sets of the two exercises below.

Dumbbell single-arm row: 7 to 8 reps/arm (use a weight you can handle for 10 to 12 reps) (rest thirty seconds)
Dumbbell single-arm overhead press: 7 to 8 reps/arm (use a weight you can handle for 10 to 12 reps) (rest two minutes)

METABOLIC CIRCUIT
Set a timer for eight minutes. Complete as many rounds of this three-exercise circuit as possible, resting as little as needed.

Dumbbell single-arm overhead press (half-kneeling): 8 reps/arm
Dumbbell chest-supported row: 12 reps
Push-up: 10 to 20 reps (can do on a bench or bar or from your knees)

Day 3: Total Body

WARM-UP
Do 10 reps each of:

Bodyweight squat
Jumping jacks
Bodyweight row
Bodyweight lunge
Inchworm

Try to cycle through at least two to three times and let the fun begin.

METABOLIC CIRCUIT
First, do two warm-up sets of only three reps each with a light weight. Then perform five rounds of this four-exercise complex. Try to use the same weight you used last week (or heavier, if you can hit all the reps). Try to rest as little as possible between each exercise. If possible, go from one exercise to the next, but feel free to rest if you need to catch your breath and then push hard again.

Dumbbell overhead press: 8 reps
Dumbbell Romanian deadlift: 8 reps
Dumbbell bent-over row: 8 reps
Dumbbell squat: 8 reps

Day 4: Total Body

WARM-UP

Perform five reps on each side of this one incredible move. It might take a few reps to get the hang of it, but it'll loosen up your entire body and have you ready to train.

World's greatest stretch: 5 rounds per side

METABOLIC CIRCUIT

Set a timer for twenty-five minutes. Do the first exercise for thirty seconds, then rest for thirty seconds. Cycle through each exercise until time is up. When you finish, start over at the beginning.

Dumbbell reverse lunge (alternating)

Push-up

Dumbbell squat

Hollow body hold

Bodyweight single-leg Romanian deadlift (left leg)

Dumbbell bent-over row

Bodyweight single-leg Romanian deadlift (right leg)

Dumbbell squat + overhead press

Week 2: Bodyweight Workout

Day 1: Lower Body

WARM-UP

Hip raise: 2 sets x 12 reps

Bodyweight lunge: 2 sets x 12 reps/leg

Dead bug: 2 sets x 8 reps/side

STRENGTH

Perform two to three warm-up sets of 5 to 6 reps of the exercise below (squats). Then, complete two sets of the exercises below. Rest about two minutes between sets.

Bodyweight squat: 10 to 20 reps with a four-second hold at the bottom (rest thirty seconds)

Do a bodyweight squat. As you reach the bottom of the movement, stay in the squat position for four seconds (also called a four-second isometric hold), then stand back up. The goal minimum reps is 10. The maximum is 20. Do what works for your fitness level.

Step-up: 10 reps/leg (rest two minutes after you do all reps)

METABOLIC CIRCUIT

Set a timer for eight minutes. Complete as many rounds of this three-exercise circuit as possible, resting as little as needed.

Bodyweight lunge (alternating): 10 reps/leg
Plank (if you can, do alternating shoulder taps): 25 seconds
Bodyweight split squat: 15 reps/leg

Front foot can be elevated a few inches off the floor (think of standing on a phone book . . . if you don't know what a phone book is, clearly I'm just old).

Day 2: Upper Body

WARM-UP
Kneeling reach through to rotation: 2 sets x 6 reps/side
Inchworm: 2 sets x 8 reps
T-Superman: 2 sets x 6 reps/side

STRENGTH
Perform two to three warm-up sets of 5 to 6 reps with a light weight. Then complete two sets of the two exercises below.

Bodyweight row *or* T-Superman: 10 to 15 reps + hold one-second at the top of the movement (squeezing shoulder blades together) (rest thirty seconds)

Push-up: 10 to 20 reps + hold one-second at the top of the movement (think about pressing through your palms and separating your shoulder blades at the top)

Rest two minutes

METABOLIC CIRCUIT
Set a timer for eight minutes. Complete as many rounds of this three-exercise circuit as possible, resting as little as needed.

Band pull-apart: 10 to 15 reps
Dumbbell single-arm row (use a band instead of weights): 10 to 20 reps
Dumbbell single-arm overhead press (bodyweight okay): 10 to 20 reps

Day 3: Total Body

WARM-UP
Do 10 reps each of:

Bodyweight squat
Jumping jacks
Push-up
Bodyweight lunge
Inchworm

Cycle through two to three times and let the fun begin.

METABOLIC CIRCUIT
First, do two warm-up sets of only 3 reps each with a light weight. Then, perform five rounds of this four-exercise complex.

Dumbbell overhead press (use a band instead of weights): 12 reps
Dumbbell single-leg Romanian deadlift (bodyweight okay): 10 reps/leg
Band seated row: 12 to 20 reps
Bodyweight squat: 12 to 20 reps

Day 4: Total Body

WARM-UP
Perform 5 reps on each side of this one incredible move. It might take a few

reps to get the hang of it, but it'll loosen up your entire body and have you ready to train.

World's greatest stretch: 5 rounds per side

METABOLIC CIRCUIT

Set a timer for twenty-five minutes. Do the first exercise for thirty seconds, then rest for thirty seconds. Cycle through each exercise, starting at the beginning when you finish, until time is up.

Bodyweight lunge (alternating)
Push-up
Bodyweight squat
Hollow body hold
Bodyweight single-leg Romanian deadlift (left leg)
Mountain climber
Bodyweight single-leg Romanian deadlift (right leg)
Superman

Week 3 Workouts

This week, you'll see slight changes to your steps goal (don't forget to make that a focus!) and progressions with the training.

The goal is still three to four workouts. We're building habits that can last for a lifetime.

You can schedule the workouts as you want, but—ideally—you won't train on back-to-back days. That said, it's easier to do day one and day two back-to-back. Whereas, if you can, try to have a day of rest between workout three and workout four. Otherwise, simply follow the approach that's outlined for each day.

This week, aim for a minimum of 7,000 steps every day. This makes a big difference for many health benefits. Don't underestimate its power.

Every workout is still in the twenty- to thirty-minute range. Keep thinking, *intensity*. With this plan, every set counts. Even your warm-ups—when the weight is lower—should be done with intention and focus on the movement. I want you to push each set hard, but at a weight you feel in complete control of every rep.

Week 3: Weight/Equipment Workout

Day 1: Lower Body

Little changes, big results: The adjustments below might seem subtle, but they can be substantial. Let's say you're using the example above and your working sets are 20 pounds on both exercises (note that you don't need to use the same weight on both exercises). Imagine last week you did 7 reps with 20 pounds. This week, the goal is 9 reps on each exercise. Doesn't seem like much, right? But, just do the math:

Last week

7 reps x 20 pounds = 140 pounds/set
2 sets total x 140 pounds = 280 pounds per exercise
2 exercises total x 280 pounds/exercise = 560 pounds lifted

This week

9 reps x 20 pounds = 180 pounds/set
2 sets total x 180 pounds = 360 pounds per exercise
2 exercises total x 360 pounds/exercise = 720 pounds

Look! With just two extra reps per set, you've increased your total workload by 160 pounds! That's how results happen.

WARM-UP
Hip raise: 2 sets x 15 reps
Bodyweight lunge: 2 sets x 15 reps/leg
Dead bug: 2 sets x 12 reps/side

STRENGTH
First, perform two to three warm-up sets of both exercises with a light weight. Then, do one exercise, rest thirty seconds, and then do the next exercise. Complete two sets.

Goblet squat: 9 to 10 reps (use a weight you can sustain for 10 to 12 reps) (rest thirty seconds)

Dumbbell Romanian deadlift: 9 to 10 reps (use a weight you can sustain for 10 to 12 reps) (rest two minutes and then repeat)

METABOLIC CIRCUIT
Set a timer for ten minutes (we're adding two minutes this week). Complete as many rounds of this three-exercise circuit as possible, resting as little as needed.

Dumbbell reverse lunge (alternating): 8 reps/leg
Plank row: 12 reps/arm
Step-up (bodyweight or dumbbell): 15 reps

Day 2: Upper Body

WARM-UP
Kneeling reach through to rotation: 2 sets x 8 reps/side
Inchworm: 2 sets x 10 reps
Band pull-apart: 2 sets x 12 to 15 reps

STRENGTH
First, perform two to three warm-up sets with a light weight. Then, complete two sets of the two exercises below.

Dumbbell single-arm row: 9 to 10 reps/arm (use a weight you can sustain for 10 to 12 reps) (rest thirty seconds)
Dumbbell single-arm overhead press: 9 to 10 reps/arm (use a weight you can sustain for 10 to 12 reps) (rest two minutes)

METABOLIC CIRCUIT
Set a timer for ten minutes (again, adding two more minutes). Complete as many rounds of this three-exercise circuit as possible, resting as little as needed.

Dumbbell single-arm overhead press (half-kneeling): 8 reps/arm
Dumbbell chest-supported row: 12 reps
Push-up: 10 to 20 reps (can do on a bench or bar or from your knees)

Day 3: Total Body

WARM-UP
Do 10 reps each of:

Bodyweight squat
Jumping jacks
Bodyweight row
Dumbbell reverse lunge (bodyweight)
Inchworm

Cycle through two to three times and let the fun begin.

METABOLIC CIRCUIT
Perform six rounds of this four-exercise complex. This week, we're adding an additional round *and* one more rep to each exercise. Remember, these small changes add up to *a lot*.

First, do two warm-up sets of only 3 reps each using a light weight. Then, trying to use the same weight you used last week (or heavier, if you can hit all the reps) and resting as little as possible between each exercise, go from one exercise to the next. If you need to, feel free to rest and catch your breath so you can push hard.

Dumbbell overhead press: 9 reps
Dumbbell Romanian deadlift: 9 reps
Dumbbell bent-over row: 9 reps
Dumbbell squat: 9 reps

Day 4: Total Body

WARM-UP
Perform 6 reps on each side of this one incredible move. It might take a few reps to get the hang of it, but it'll loosen up your entire body and have you ready to train.

World's greatest stretch: 6 rounds per side

METABOLIC CIRCUIT

Set a timer for twenty-five minutes. Do the first exercise for forty seconds, then rest for twenty seconds. You're adding ten seconds of work and removing ten seconds of rest. Cycle through each movement, starting at the beginning when you finish, until time is up.

Dumbbell reverse lunge (alternating)
Push-up
Dumbbell squat
Hollow body hold
Dumbbell single-leg Romanian deadlift (left leg)
Bent-over dumbbell row
Dumbbell single-leg Romanian deadlift (right leg)
Dumbbell squat + overhead press

Week 3: Bodyweight Workouts

Day 1: Lower Body

WARM-UP
Hip raise: 2 sets x 15 reps
Dumbbell reverse lunge (bodyweight okay): 2 sets x 12 to 15 reps/leg
Dead bug: 2 sets x 10 reps/side

STRENGTH
Perform two to three warm-up sets of 5 to 6 reps of the exercise below (squats). Then, complete two sets of the exercises below. Rest for about two minutes between sets.

Bodyweight squat: 15 to 25 reps with a four-second hold at the bottom (rest thirty seconds)
Perform a bodyweight squat. As you reach the bottom of the movement, stay in the squat position for four seconds (also called a four-second isometric hold), then stand back up. The goal minimum is 15 reps. The maximum is 25. Do what works for your fitness level.
Step-up: 12 reps/leg (then rest for two minutes)

METABOLIC CIRCUIT

Set a timer for ten minutes. Complete as many rounds of this three-exercise circuit as possible, resting as little as needed.

Dumbbell reverse lunge (alternating): 10 reps/leg
Plank (if you can, do alternating shoulder-taps): 25 seconds
Dumbbell split squat: 15 reps/leg
Your front foot can be elevated a few inches off the floor

Day 2: Upper Body

WARM-UP

Kneeling reach through to rotation: 2 sets x 8 reps/side
Inchworm: 2 sets x 10 reps
T-Superman:: 2 sets x 8 reps/side
(If you can't do a push-up, just do T-rotations, which is the same movement but without the push-up)

STRENGTH

Perform two to three warm-up sets of 5 to 6 reps. Then, complete two sets of the two exercises below.

Bodyweight row *or* T-superman: 15 to 20 reps + hold one-second at the top of the movement (squeezing shoulder blades together) (rest thirty seconds)
Push-up: 15 to 25 reps + hold one-second at the top of the movement (think about pressing through your palms and separating your shoulder blades at the top) (rest two minutes)

METABOLIC CIRCUIT

Set a timer for ten minutes. Complete as many rounds of this three-exercise circuit as possible, resting as little as needed.

Band pull-apart: 10 to 15 reps
Dumbbell single-arm row (with a band instead of weights): 10 to 20 reps
Dumbbell single-arm overhead press: 10 to 20 reps

Day 3: Total Body

WARM-UP
Do ten reps each of:

Bodyweight squat
Jumping jacks
Push-up
Dumbbell reverse lunge (bodyweight okay)
Inchworm

Cycle through two to three times and let the fun begin.

METABOLIC CIRCUIT
First, do two warm-up sets of only 3 reps each with a light weight. Then, perform six rounds of this four-exercise complex.

Dumbbell overhead press (with a band instead of weights): 15 reps
Bodyweight single-leg Romanian deadlift: 12 reps/leg
Bodyweight row (seated, with a band): 12 to 20 reps
Bodyweight squat: 12 to 20 reps

Day 4: Total Body

WARM-UP
Perform six reps on each side of this one incredible move. It might take a few reps to get the hang of it, but it'll loosen up your entire body and have you ready to train.

World's greatest stretch: 6 rounds per side

METABOLIC CIRCUIT
Set a timer for twenty-five minutes. Do the first exercise for forty seconds, then rest for twenty seconds. Cycle through each movement, starting again at the top when you finish, until time is up.

Dumbbell reverse lunge (alternating)
Push-up
Bodyweight squat
Hollow body hold
Bodyweight single-leg Romanian deadlift (left leg)
Mountain climber
Bodyweight single-leg Romanian deadlift (right leg)
Superman

Week 4 Workouts

Once again, complete three to four workouts each week. If you do only three workouts in a week, start the following week with workout four, and then begin the next sequence of workouts.

Once again, try to get a minimum of 7,000 steps every day.

It's going to look familiar, but now it's time to measure the progress you've made. The program is basically the same as week one, but you should now be stronger, have better endurance, and be capable of pushing yourself harder than just a few weeks ago.

Week 4: Weight/Equipment Workout

Day 1: Lower Body

WARM-UP
Hip raise: 2 sets x 12 reps
Dumbbell reverse lunge (bodyweight okay): 2 sets x 12 reps/leg
Dead bug: 2 sets x 8 reps/side

STRENGTH
First, perform two to three warm-up sets with a light weight. Then, complete three to four sets of the exercises below.

Goblet squat: 5 to 6 reps (use a weight you can sustain for 7 to 8 reps)
Dumbbell Romanian deadlift: 5 to 6 reps (use a weight you can sustain for 7 to 8 reps)

METABOLIC CIRCUIT

Set a timer for eight minutes. Complete as many rounds of this three-exercise circuit as possible, resting as little as needed. You're likely using more weight now (or completing more rounds) than when you started.

Dumbbell reverse lunge (alternating): 8 reps/leg
Plank row: 12 reps/arm
Step-up (bodyweight or dumbbell): 15 reps

Day 2: Upper Body

WARM-UP

Kneeling reach through to rotation: 2 sets x 6 reps/side
Inchworm: 2 sets x 8 reps
Band pull-apart: 2 sets x 10 reps

STRENGTH

First, perform two to three warm-up sets using a light weight. Then, complete three to four sets of the exercise below.

Single-arm row: 5 to 6 reps/arm (use a weight you can sustain for 7 to 8 reps)
Single-arm overhead press: 5 to 6 reps/arm (use a weight you can sustain for 7 to 8 reps)

METABOLIC CIRCUIT

Set a timer for eight minutes. Complete as many rounds of this three-exercise circuit as possible, resting as little as needed.

Dumbbell overhead press: 8 reps
Dumbbell chest-supported row: 12 reps
Push-up: as many as possible (can do on a bench or bar or from your knees)

Day 3: Total Body

WARM-UP

Set a timer for three minutes and do 10 reps each of:

Bodyweight squat
Jumping jacks
Bodyweight row
Bodyweight reverse lunge (bodyweight okay)
Inchworm

Cycle through two to three times and let the fun begin.

METABOLIC CIRCUIT

First, do two warm-up sets of only 3 reps each with a light weight. Then, perform six rounds of this four-exercise complex. Ideally, you're using more weight than you did in week one. Remember, you've built both strength and endurance. After doing 10 reps/exercise last week, six reps will feel very different.

Dumbbell overhead press: 6 reps
Dumbbell Romanian deadlift: 6 reps
Dumbbell bent-over row: 6 reps
Dumbbell squat: 6 reps

Day 4: Total Body

WARM-UP

Perform five reps on each side of this one incredible move. It might take a few reps to get the hang of it, but it'll loosen up your entire body and have you ready to train.

Squat strider kick-through flow: 5 rounds per side

STRENGTH-METABOLIC CIRCUIT

Set a timer for twenty-five minutes. Do the first exercise for twenty seconds, then rest for forty seconds. You've flipped back to the initial twenty seconds of work, so you can use heavier weights because it's a more intense, shorter work period (and longer rest). Repeat, cycling through each exercise, until time is up. Start back at the beginning if you finish.

Dumbbell reverse lunge (alternating)
Push-up

Dumbbell squat
Hollow body hold
Bodyweight single-leg Romanian deadlift (left leg)
Dumbbell bent-over row
Bodyweight single-leg Romanian deadlift (right leg)
Dumbbell squat + overhead press

Week 4: Bodyweight Workouts

Day 1: Lower Body

WARM-UP
Hip raise: 2 sets x 15 reps
Dumbbell reverse lunge (bodyweight): 2 sets x 12 to 15 reps/leg
Dead bug: 2 sets x 10 reps/side

STRENGTH
Perform two to three warm-up sets of 5 to 6 reps of the exercise below
(squats). Then, complete two sets of the exercises below. Rest for about two
minutes between sets.

Bodyweight squat: 20 to 30 reps with a four-second hold at the bottom (rest
thirty seconds)
Perform a bodyweight squat. As you reach the bottom of the movement, stay
in the squat position for four seconds (also called a four-second isometric hold),
then stand back up. The goal minimum is 15 reps. The maximum is 25. Do what
works for your fitness level.
Step-up: 15 reps/leg (rest two minutes after you do all reps)

METABOLIC CIRCUIT
Set a timer for eight minutes. Complete as many rounds of this three-exercise
circuit as possible, resting as little as needed.

Dumbbell reverse lunge (alternating): 8 reps/leg
Plank (if you can, do alternating shoulder-taps): 20 seconds
Step-up: 15 reps

Day 2: Upper Body

WARM-UP
Kneeling reach through to rotation: 2 sets x 8 reps/side
Inchworm: 2 sets x 10 reps
T-Superman: 2 sets x 8 reps/side
(If you can't do a push-up, just do T-rotations, which is the same movement
but without the push-up)

STRENGTH
Perform two to three warm-up sets of 5 to 6 reps. Then, complete two sets of
the two exercises below.

Bodyweight row *or* T-superman: 20 to 25 reps + hold one-second at the top of
the movement (squeezing shoulder blades together) (rest thirty seconds)
Push-up: 20 to 30 reps + hold one-second at the top of the movement (think
about pressing through your palms and separating your shoulder blades at the
top) (rest two minutes)

METABOLIC CIRCUIT
Set a timer for eight minutes. Complete as many rounds of this three-exercise
circuit as possible, resting as little as needed.

Band pull apart: 10 to 15 reps
Dumbbell single-arm row (with a band instead of weights): 10 to 20 reps
Push-up: 10 to 20 reps (can do on a bench or bar or from your knees)

Day 3: Total Body

WARM-UP
Do 10 reps each of:

Bodyweight squat
Jumping jacks
Push-up
Dumbbell reverse lunge (bodyweight okay)
Inchworm

Cycle through two to three times and let the fun begin.

METABOLIC CIRCUIT

Do two warm-up sets of only 3 reps each. Then perform eight rounds of this four-exercise complex.

Dumbbell overhead press (with a band instead of weights): 12 reps
Bodyweight single-leg Romanian deadlift: 12 reps/leg
Bodyweight row (seated, with a band): 15 reps
Bodyweight squat: 15 reps

Day 4: Total Body

WARM-UP

Perform six reps on each side of this one incredible move. It might take a few reps to get the hang of it, but it'll loosen up your entire body and have you ready to train.

World's greatest stretch: 6 rounds per side

Set a timer for twenty-five minutes. Do the first exercise for twenty seconds, then rest for forty seconds. Cycle through each movement until time is up, starting at the top when you finish the last exercise.

Dumbbell reverse lunge (alternating)
Push-up
Bodyweight squat
Hollow body hold
bodyweight single-leg Romanian deadlift (left leg)
Mountain climber
Bodyweight single-leg Romanian deadlift (right leg)
Superman

Week 5 Workouts

This will be a new look, but we'll progress in a similar fashion. Once again, do your best to get in your steps. Your new minimum is 7,000 steps, and your stretch goal is 10,000 steps per day. Let the fun begin!

Day 1: Full Bod

WARM-UP
Kneeling reach through to rotation: 2 sets x 6 reps/side
Dumbbell reverse lunge (alternating): 2 sets x 8 reps
Band pull apart: 2 sets x 10 reps

METABOLIC CIRCUIT
First, complete one to two warm-up sets, usually about 40% to 50% of the weight you plan to use (for push-ups, do 6 to 8 reps). Then, complete one set of the following four exercises as a "giant set," which means completing one exercise after the other with as little rest as possible. Rest two minutes and then repeat for a second round.

Goblet squat: 2 sets x 6 to 8 reps
Bodyweight arm row: 2 sets x 8 to 12 reps
Hip raise: 2 sets x 8 to 10 reps
Push-up: 2 sets x as many reps as possible

Next, complete one warm-up set, usually about 40% to 50% of the weight you plan to use. Then, complete one set of the following four exercises as a "giant set," which means completing one exercise after another with as little rest as possible. Rest two minutes and then repeat for a second round.

Lying hamstring curl (feet on Valsides, furniture sliders, or paper plates): 2 sets x 10 to 12 reps
Dumbbell single-arm overhead press: 2 sets x 6 to 8 reps
Dumbbell bent-over row (two arms): 2 sets x 6 to 8 reps
Dumbbell reverse lunge: 2 sets x 6 to 8 reps

Day 2: Full Body

WARM-UP
Kneeling reach through to rotation: 2 sets x 6 reps/side
Inchworm: 2 sets x 8 reps
Band pull-apart: 2 sets x 10 reps

METABOLIC CIRCUIT
First, complete one to two warm-up sets, usually about 40% to 50% of the weight you plan to use. Then, complete one set of the following four exercises as a "giant set," which means completing one exercise after another with as little rest as possible. Rest two minutes and then repeat for a second round.

Dumbbell reverse lunge (alternating): 2 sets x 6 to 8/leg
Dumbbell overhead press: 2 sets x 12 to 15 reps
Dumbbell kickstand Romanian deadlift: 2 sets x 10 to 15 reps/leg
Dumbbell bent-over reverse fly: 2 sets x 8 to 12 reps

Next, complete one to two warm-up sets, usually about 40% to 50% of the weight you plan to use. Then, complete one set of the following four exercises as a "giant set," which means completing one exercise after another with as little rest as possible. Rest two minutes and then repeat for a second round.

Dumbbell chest press: 2 sets x 6 to 8 reps
Dumbbell step-up: 2 sets x 6 to 8 reps/leg
Hollow body hold: 2 sets x 30 seconds
Farmer's walks: 2 sets x 30 seconds

Day 3: Dumbbell Ladder
Perform eight rounds of the following sequence. This is considered a workout "ladder." You'll do 1 rep of each exercise. Catch your breath, and then do 2 reps of each exercise. Rest again. And, then move to 3 reps. The goal is to work up to 7 reps of each exercise. Choose a weight you can normally do for 10 to 12 reps. The first couple rounds will feel easy . . . and then it'll get much harder.

WARM-UP

First, set a timer for two minutes and cycle through these exercises:

Bodyweight squat: 5 reps
Push-up plus (pressing shoulder blades apart in a plank position): 5 reps
Spiderman lunge with rotation (alternating): 5 reps
Band pull-apart: 5 reps

The ladder: Start at 1-rep of each exercise and work up to 7 reps of each exercise.

Dumbbell skier swings
Dumbbell bent-over row
Dumbbell squat
Dumbbell single-arm row (alternating)
Dumbbell reverse lunge
Dumbbell Romanian deadlift

Day 4: The Terrible Two's

The end of the week is a chance to finish strong. This workout brings the best of strength and cardio into a fast-paced action that will challenge your body in ways you'll hopefully love.

WARM-UP

Perform 5 reps on each side of this one incredible move. It might take a few reps to get the hang of it, but it'll loosen up your entire body and have you ready to train.

World's greatest stretch: 5 rounds per side

The following sequence is a circuit. First, do two warm-up sets with about 50% of the weight you'll choose.

Then, perform 2 reps of each exercise using a weight that you can lift for approximately 5 to 6 reps. Set a timer for twenty-five minutes, resting as necessary, and keep doing sets of 2 reps until the time is up.

Dumbbell *or* Barbell Romanian deadlift: 2 reps
Dumbbell single-arm *or* Barbell row: 2 reps

Dumbbell *or* Barbell Bulgarian split squat: 2 reps
Dumbbell *or* Barbell overhead press: 2 reps
Medicine ball slam: 2 reps

Week 6 Workouts

You've arrived at the final week of training! It's an amazing accomplishment, and you should be proud of the progress you've made.

Remember, after you finish this week, cycle back to week one of this program. Do a second phase, and you'll be amazed at how much stronger you've become and how replaying the program will unlock new changes and improvements to your body.

Once again, prioritize low-intensity movement. At a minimum, aim for at least 7,000 steps per day and a stretch goal of 10,000 steps per day.

Let the fun begin!

Day 1: Full Body

WARM-UP
Kneeling reach through to rotation: 2 sets x 6 reps/side
Dumbbell reverse lunge (alternating, bodyweight okay): 2 sets x 8 reps
Band pull-apart: 2 sets x 10 reps

METABOLIC CIRCUIT
First, complete 1 to 2 warm-up sets, usually about 40% to 50% of the weight you plan to use (for push-ups, do 6 to 8 reps). Then, complete one set of the following four exercises as a "giant set," which means completing one exercise after another with as little rest as possible. Rest two minutes and then repeat for a second round.

Goblet squat: 2 sets x 10 to 12 reps
Dumbbell single-arm row: 2 sets x 12 to 15 reps
Hip raise: 2 sets x 10 to 12 reps
Push-up: 2 sets x as many reps as possible.

Next, complete one warm-up set, usually about 40% to 50% of the weight you plan to use. Then, complete one set of the following four exercises as a "giant set," which means completing one exercise after another with as little rest as possible. Rest two minutes and then repeat for a second round.

Lying hamstring curl (feet on Valsides, furniture sliders, or paper plates): 2 sets x 12 to 15 reps

Dumbbell single-arm overhead press: 2 sets x 10 to 12 reps

Dumbbell bent-over row: 2 sets x 10 to 12 reps

Dumbbell reverse lunge: 2 sets x 10 to 12 reps

Day 2: Full Body

WARM-UP

Kneeling reach through to rotation: 2 sets x 6 reps/side

Inchworm: 2 sets x 8 reps

Band pull-apart: 2 sets x 10 reps

First, complete one to two warm-up sets, usually about 40% to 50% of the weight you plan to use. Then, complete one set of the following four exercises as a "giant set," which means completing one exercise after another with as little rest as possible. Rest two minutes and then repeat for a second round.

Dumbbell reverse lunge (alternating): 2 sets x 8 to 10/leg

Dumbbell overhead press: 2 sets x 15 to 20 reps

Dumbbell kickstand Romanian deadlift: 2 sets x 15 to 20 reps/leg

Dumbbell bent-over reverse fly: 2 sets x 12 to 15 reps

Next, complete one to two warm-up sets, usually about 40% to 50% of the weight you plan to use. Then, complete one set of the following four exercises as a "giant set," which means completing one exercise after another with as little rest as possible. Rest two minutes and then repeat for a second round.

Dumbbell chest press: 2 sets x 10 to 12 reps

Dumbbell step-up: 2 sets x 10 to 12 reps/leg

Hollow body hold: 2 sets x 30 seconds (hold weight overhead if you want to make harder)

Farmer's walks: 2 sets x 30 seconds (grab heavier weights)

Day 3: Dumbbell Ladder

Perform eight rounds of the following sequence. This is considered a workout "ladder." You'll do 1 rep of each exercise. Catch your breath, and then do 2 reps of each exercise. Rest again. And, then move to 3 reps. The goal is to work up to 8 reps of each exercise. Choose a weight you can normally do for 10 to 12 reps. The first couple rounds will feel easy . . . and then it'll get much harder.

This week, try to add a little bit of weight compared to the prior week, even if just 5 pounds.

WARM-UP

First, set a timer for two minutes and cycle through the following exercises:

Bodyweight squat: 5 reps

Push-up plus (pressing shoulder blades apart in a plank position): 5 reps

Spiderman lunge with rotation (alternating): 5 reps

Band pull-aparts: 5 reps

The ladder:

Dumbbell skier swings

Dumbbell bent-over row

Dumbbell squat

Dumbbell single-arm row (alternating)

Dumbbell reverse lunge

Dumbbell Romanian deadlift

Day 4: The Terrible Twos

The end of the week is a chance to finish strong. This workout brings the best of strength and cardio into a fast-paced action that will challenge your body in ways you'll hopefully love.

WARM-UP

Perform 5 reps on each side of this one incredible move. It might take a few reps to get the hang of it, but it'll loosen up your entire body and have you ready to train.

World's greatest stretch: 5 rounds per side

The following sequence is a circuit. First, do two warm-up sets with about 50% of the weight you'll choose.

Next, perform 3 reps of each exercise using a weight that you can lift for approximately 5 to 6 reps. Set a timer for twenty-five minutes, resting as necessary, and keep doing sets of 2 reps until the time is up.

Dumbbell *or* Barbell Romanian deadlift: 3 reps

Dumbbell single-arm *or* Barbell row: 3 reps

Dumbbell *or* Barbell Bulgarian split squat: 3 reps

Dumbbell *or* Barbell overhead press: 3 reps

Medicine ball slam: 3 reps

Exercise Descriptions

Use the following tips to perform the exercises in this program safely and effectively. If you'd like to see video demonstrations, visit youtube.com/Bornfitness.

Band Overhead Press

Hold one end of the band in each hand. Bend over and step on the center of the band with one foot. Stand up and hold each end of the band just outside your shoulders, your arms bent . With your knees slightly bent, press both hands up directly above your shoulders until your arms are straight, then return to the starting position.

Band Pull-Apart

Grab a band and hold your arms in front of your body at chest height. With your hands about shoulder-width apart, keep your arms straight and pull the resistance band apart by extending both arms to either side. Your body should form the letter "T." Pause, and return to the starting position.

Band Seated Row

Hold one end of the band in each hand. Sit down and loop the center of the band around the ball of your feet. Sit up tall with your legs straight. Pull the band toward your body by driving your elbows back. Stop when your hands are aligned with your ribcage, pause, and then slowly return to the starting position.

Band Single-Arm Row

Anchor a band around a fixed object, such as a door handle. Ideally, it will be around hip height. Grab the opposite end of the band (or the handle, if your band has one), and step way until there is tension in the band. Stand in a staggered stance with your knees slightly bent. Pull the band toward your body by driving your elbow back. Stop when your hand is aligned with your ribcage, pause, and then slowly return to the starting position. Do all reps and then repeat with your other arm.

Barbell Bulgarian Split Squat

Place a barbell on your upper back with an overhand grip like you were going to do a squat. Place the top of your left foot on a bench directly behind you and lower your hips until your right knee hits a 90-degree angle. Push through your right heel back to the starting position. Repeat until you accomplish the prescribed number of reps, then switch legs.

Barbell Overhead Press

Hold a barbell at shoulder height, your hands shoulder-width apart, with your arms bent and palms facing forward. Set your feet at shoulder width and bend your knees slightly. Press the barbell over your head up until your arms are straight, then return to the starting position.

Barbell Romanian Deadlift

Stand with feet shoulder-width apart and hold a barbell in front of you. Bend your knees slightly and bend at your waist with your back straight. Avoid rounding the upper back and keep your head neutral. Extend your arms fully so each dumbbell is just above the floor. Contract your back and pull both dumbbells up to your ribcage. Be sure to pull through the elbow and hold for one second in the top position. Lower the dumbbells to the fully extended arm position and repeat.

Barbell Row

Stand with feet shoulder width apart and hold a barbell in front of you. Bend your knees slightly and bend at your waist with your back straight. Avoid rounding the upper back and keep your head neutral. Extend your arms fully so each dumbbell is just above the floor. Contract your back and pull both dumbbells up to your ribcage. Be sure to pull through the elbow and hold for one second in the top position. Lower the barbell to the fully extended arm position and repeat.

Bodyweight Split Squat

Stand upright and then take a long stride forward so you're in a staggered stance with one foot in from of the other and your hands by your sides looking straight ahead. Lower your torso toward the floor by bending knees simultaneously. Lower until your back knee almost touches the ground, directly beneath your hip. Think about moving like an elevator (up and down). Pause at the bottom, and then drive through the heel of your front foot and rise back up to return to the starting position. Repeat for the desired number of repetitions on one leg, then switch the leg that is in front, and repeat.

Bodyweight Lunge

Stand tall with your feet hip-width apart. Step forward with your right leg and slowly lower your body until your front knee is bent at least 90 degrees. Don't allow the weight to carry you forward. Your rear knee should nearly touch the floor. Keep your torso as upright as possible, pause, then push yourself back up to the starting position. Then, repeat the movement, but this time by stepping forward with your left leg.

Bodyweight Reverse Lunge

Stand tall with your feet hip-width apart. Step backward with your right leg and slowly lower your body until your front knee is bent at least 90 degrees. Your rear knee should nearly touch the floor. Keep your torso as upright as possible, pause, then push yourself back up to the starting position. Then, repeat the movement, but this time by stepping backward with your left leg.

Bodyweight Row

Set a barbell at about hip height. Lie underneath the barbell and grab it with both arms. Your body should form a straight line from your shoulders to your ankles. Start the movement by retracting your shoulder blades and continue to pull while keeping your elbows next to your sides. Pause for one second at the top and return so the arms are fully extended.

Bodyweight Single-Leg Romanian Deadlift

Stand on one leg, with your arms straight and your standing leg slightly bent. Push your hips backward, lowering your torso toward the ground as your rear leg trails behind you to help with balance. Only go as low as you can without your lower back rounding. Pause, and then reverse the movement, returning to the starting position. Squeeze your glutes at the top. Do all the reps, then switch legs.

Bodyweight Squat

Stand with feet slightly wider than hip width, toes pointed straight ahead or slightly outward. Hold your arms straight out from your shoulders (parallel to the ground) and keep your head neutral, focusing on a point on the ground several feet in front of you can help. Push your hips back and lower into a squat. Keep the back neutral and core tight. Pause, and then press through your heels to stand up.

Dead Bug

Lie on your back with your legs straight up in the air. Brace your abs and keep your head and shoulders on the ground. Keep the neutral arch in your lower back and lower one leg straight toward the floor. Keep your opposite leg in the air. Return the leg to the starting position. Do all reps, switch legs, and repeat.

Dumbbell Bent-Over Reverse Fly

Stand with feet shoulder-width apart and hold a dumbbell in each hand. Bend the knees slightly and bend at the waist with your back straight. Avoid rounding the upper back and keep your head neutral. Extend your arms fully so each dumbbell is just above the floor. Keeping a slight bend in your elbows, slowly bring the dumbbells out to your sides until your arms form a "T" with your torso. Pause, then lower your arms back to the starting position.

Dumbbell Bent-Over Row

Stand with feet shoulder-width apart and hold a dumbbell in each hand. Bend the knees slightly and bend at the waist with your back straight. Avoid rounding the upper back and keep your head neutral. Extend your arms fully so each dumbbell is just above the floor. Contract your back and pull both dumbbells up to your ribcage. Be sure to pull through the elbow and hold for one second in the top position. Lower the dumbbells to the fully extended arm position and repeat.

Dumbbell Bulgarian Split Squat

Grab a dumbbell in each hand. Place the top of your left foot on a bench directly behind you and lower your hips until your right knee hits a 90-degree angle. Push through your right heel back to the starting position. Repeat until you accomplish the prescribed number of reps, and then switch legs.

Dumbbell Chest Press

Grasp a pair of dumbbells. Lie on your back on a bench and hold the dumbbells over your chest. (If you don't have a bench, you can still perform the movement from the floor.) Pull the dumbbells down toward your chest, pause, and then press the weights back up to the starting position.

Dumbbell Chest-Supported Row

Set a bench to about a 45-degree angle. Grab a pair of dumbbells and lean into the bench with your face looking at the floor. (If you don't have a bench, slightly bend your knees and bend at your waist so that your torso is at a 45-degree angle to the floor. Then, perform reps as described.) With both of your arms extending, pull the dumbbells up toward your chest and squeeze your shoulder blades together. Pause, then lower the dumbbells back to the starting position.

Dumbbell Kickstand Romanian Deadlift

Grab two dumbbells and hold them at your sides. Stand in a staggered stance with your front leg firmly planted on the floor and your back foot pressing through your toes (your heel will be off the floor). Push your hips backward and feel the tension in the back of your leg. Only go as low as you can without your lower back rounding. Pause, then reverse the movement, returning to the starting position. Squeeze your glutes at the top. Do all the reps, then switch legs.

Dumbbell Overhead Press

Hold a pair of dumbbells just outside your shoulders, your arms bent and palms facing each other. Set your feet at shoulder width and bend your knees slightly. Press both dumbbells up until your arms are straight, then return to the starting position.

Dumbbell Reverse Lunge

Grab a pair of dumbbells and hold them at arm's length next to your sides, your palms facing each other. Step backward with your right leg and slowly lower your body until your front knee is bent at least 90 degrees. Pause, then push yourself to the starting position as quickly as you can. Complete the prescribed number of reps with your right leg, then do the same number with your left leg.

Dumbbell Romanian Deadlift

Grab two dumbbells and hold them at your sides. Push your hips backward, lowering your torso toward the ground, only going as low as you can without rounding your lower back. Pause, then reverse the movement, returning to the starting position. Squeeze your glutes at the top.

Dumbbell Single-Arm Overhead Press

Hold one dumbbell just outside your shoulder with your arm bent and your palm facing your head. Set your feet at shoulder width and bend your knees slightly. Press the dumbbell up until your arm is straight, then return to the starting position. Do all the reps, grab the dumbbell in your other hand, and repeat.

Dumbbell Single-Arm Row

Place a dumbbell on the floor. Bend at your hips (don't round your lower back) and lower your torso until it's almost parallel to the floor. Grab the dumbbell and let it hang at arm's length from your shoulder. Without moving your torso, row the dumbbell upward by raising your upper arms, bending your elbows, and squeezing your shoulder blades together. Pause, then lower the dumbbell back to start. Do all the reps, switch the dumbbell to your other hand, and repeat.

Dumbbell Single-Leg Romanian Deadlift

Grab two dumbbells and hold them at your sides. Stand on one leg with your arms straight and your standing leg slightly bent, push your hips backward, lowering your torso toward the ground as your rear leg trails behind you to help with balance. Only go as low as you can without your lower back rounding. Pause, then reverse the movement, returning to the starting position. Squeeze your glutes at the top. Do all the reps, then switch legs.

Dumbbell Skier Swings

Hold a pair of dumbbells at arm's length next to your thighs. Start in a strong athletic base, feet hip-to-shoulder-width apart with a slight bend in your knees. Next, swing the dumbbells behind you while pushing your hips and hamstrings back as far as you can. Do this until your trunk is parallel with the floor while keeping your knees soft and a slight natural arch in your back. Explosively thrust your hips forward and come to a full stand, squeezing your glutes at the top of the movement. At the same time, swing your arms forward until they're in front of your chest. That's 1 rep.

Dumbbell Split Squat

Stand upright holding a dumbbell in each hand. Take a long stride forward so you're in a staggered stance with one foot in from of the other and your hands by your sides looking straight ahead. Lower your torso toward the floor by bending knees simultaneously. Lower until your back knee almost touches the ground, directly beneath your hip. Think about moving like an elevator (up and down). Pause at the bottom, and then drive through the heel of your front foot and rise back up to return to the starting position. Repeat for the desired number of repetitions on one leg, then switch the leg that is in front, and repeat.

Dumbbell Squat

Stand with your feet shoulder-width apart. Hold a pair of dumbbells so that your palms are facing each other, and rest one of the dumbbell heads on the meatiest part of each shoulder. Keep your body as upright as you can at all times, with your upper arms parallel to the floor. Brace your abs and lower your body as far as you can by pushing your hips back and bending your knees. Pause, then push yourself back to the starting position.

Dumbbell Squat + Overhead Press

Stand with your feet shoulder-width apart. Hold a pair of dumbbells so that your palms are facing each other at shoulder height. Keep your body as upright as you can at all times, with your upper arms parallel to the floor. Brace your abs and lower your body as far as you can by pushing your hips back and bending your knees. Pause, then push yourself back to the starting position and then press the dumbbells overhead until your arms almost completely straight. Lower your arms back down. That's 1 rep.

Dumbbell Step-Up

Hold a dumbbell in each hand and stand a few inches away from a step or bench. Place one foot on top of the step, with your heel flat on it. Step up, keeping your torso tall. Brace your core and straighten your leg to bring yourself to standing on the step. Keeping your shoulders back and head up, lower your leg down slowly to the ground.

Farmer's Walk

Grab a heavy pair of dumbbells (one in each hand), and hold them at your sides with your arms straight. Keeping your torso upright and preventing your body from hunching over, slowly take one step after another and walk. Do this for the suggested time, and then put the dumbbells down and rest.

Goblet Squat

Hold a dumbbell vertically next to your chest, with both hands cupping the dumbbell head right under your chin. Your feet should be twice hip-width apart. Push your hips back and lower your body into a squat until your upper thighs are at least parallel to the floor. Your elbows should brush the insides of your knees in the bottom position. Pause, then push your body back up to the starting position.

Hip Raise

Lie on your back with your knees bent and your feet flat against the floor. Keep your feet hip-width apart. Tighten your stomach and press your heels into the floor, driving your hips up and finishing the movement by squeezing your butt, making sure not to use your lower back. Return to the starting position.

Hollow Body Hold

Lie on your back with arms fully extended overhead and hands together. Position your feet against each other. Brace your core and simultaneously raise your arms and legs off the ground. Hold this position by squeezing your abs and glutes.

Inchworm

Stand tall with your legs straight. Bend over to touch the floor and place your hands on the ground (slightly bend your knees if you have to). Walk your hands forward while keeping your legs straight so that you almost end up in a push-up position. Walk your feet forward in small steps with your hands on the ground so that you end up in the starting position. Repeat.

Jumping Jacks

Stand with your feet together and your hands at your sides. Simultaneously raise your arms above your head and jump your feet out to the sides. Immediately, reverse the movement and jump back to the starting position. Repeat for all reps.

Kneeling Reach Through

Start on all fours, with your hands directly under your shoulders and your back flat. Lift your right hand off the floor, and rotate your body so that your chest is facing the ceiling, as you raise your arm up in the air. Rotate your body back down toward the starting position, but—instead of returning your hand to the floor, rotate your chest toward your opposite shoulder and extend your arm across your body. It should look like you're "threading the needle" by putting your right arm under your left shoulder. Rotate back and return to the starting position. Then, repeat the movement with your other arm.

Lying Hamstring Curl

Lie on your back with your hands by your sides, knees bent, and heels on paper plates or furniture sliders. Raise your hips by pressing through your heels, then pull both legs toward your butt while keeping your hips up. You should feel the muscles in the back of your legs working. Pause and return to the starting position

Medicine Ball Slam

Grab a light medicine ball (think six to eight pounds) and hold it above your head. Your arms should be slightly bent and your feet shoulder-width apart. Forcefully slam the ball to the floor in front of you as hard as you can. Pick up the ball and repeat. Perform all reps.

Mountain Climber

Start in the push-up position with your arms completely straight and directly beneath your shoulders. Your body should form a straight line from your shoulders to your ankles. Squeeze your abs, lift one foot off the floor and bring your knee up toward your chest while keeping your body in as straight of a line as possible. Return to the starting position and repeat the movement with your opposite leg.

Plank

Lie face down with your elbows directly beneath your shoulders and press your body up into push-up position. Your body should form a straight line from your shoulders to your ankles. Tighten your abs, squeeze your butt, and hold this position for the desired amount of time.

Plank Row

Get into the top of a push-up position, but instead of your hands being placed on the floor, grip two dumbbells with your palms facing each other. Make sure that your arms are completely straight and your hands are directly beneath your shoulders. Keeping your stomach tight and elbows close to your body, row one dumbbell off the ground, pulling your elbow as high as you can while you squeeze your shoulder blade back. Return the dumbbell to the floor and repeat with your other arm.

Plank Shoulder Taps

Lie face down with your elbows directly beneath your shoulders and press your body up into push-up position. Your body should form a straight line from your shoulders to your ankles. Tighten your abs, squeeze your butt, and hold this position. Then, lift your right hand off the floor, touch your left shoulder, and then return your hand back to the floor. Repeat with your left hand touching your right shoulder. Complete for the prescribed reps.

Push-Up

Begin in the standard push-up position with your body forming a straight line from your ankles to your shoulders. Lower your body toward the floor and stop before your chest touches. Pause, then press your body back to the starting position.

Push-Up Plus

Begin in a push-up position. Your body should form a straight line from your ankles to your shoulders. Squeeze your abs as tight as possible and keep them contracted for the entire exercise. Lower your body until your chest nearly touches the floor. Pause, then push yourself back to the starting position. Once your arms are fully extended, continue pressing your palms into the ground and drive your shoulder blades toward the ceiling. Pause, then repeat the entire movement.

Spiderman Lunge with Rotation

Start in a plank position with your hands directly underneath your shoulders. Brace your core, squeeze your glutes, and engage your shoulder blades, as you would with any other plank. From the plank position, step your right foot forward and place it outside your right hand. Hold your position for a count as you rotate your torso and reach toward the sky with your left hand. Rotate back, and then return your right leg back to its original position in the plank. Then, repeat the same movement with your left leg.

Step-Up

Stand a few inches away from a step or bench. Place one foot on top of the step, with your heel flat on it. Step up, keeping your torso tall. Brace your core and straighten your leg to bring yourself to standing on the step. Keeping your shoulders back and head up, lower your leg down slowly to the ground.

Superman

Lie facedown on a flat and stable exercise bench. Hold on to the end of the bench with your hands. The other end of the bench should be just above your waist. Bend your knees and brace your abs. Squeeze your glutes and lift your legs up. Form a straight line from your knees to your shoulders. Return your legs to the starting position. Complete all the reps.

T-Superman

Lying on your stomach, extend your hands in front of your head. Keeping your head in a neutral position and looking toward the floor, lift your arms and legs up toward the ceiling. Feel as if you're reaching far away from your body with your hands and feet.

World's Greatest Stretch

Stand with your feet together and your hands at your sides. Lift you right knee toward your chest, grasping it with both hands just below your knee-cap. Then pull it as close to the middle of your chest as you can, while you stand up tall. Release your right leg, put your foot on the floor, and step into a lunge position with your front (right) leg bent 90 degrees and your back knee touching the floor. Maintaining this position, place both of your hands on the floor. Keeping your right hand on the floor near your instep, rotate and open your torso and reach over head with your left arm until it is straight, and return your arm back to the floor. Finally, lift your back knee off the floor and start to straighten your front leg. You should feel a stretch on the backside of your right leg. Stand up, then take a step forward and repeat on your left leg.

EPILOGUE
Comfortable at Last

When the student is ready, the teacher will appear.
—*Buddha Siddhartha Guatama Shakyamuni*

THIS IS NOT GOING to go the way you think.

When people have a life-changing experience, it's rarely what they expect. If it were, you would have made the switch much sooner. I expect this to be a similar eye-opening experience. After all, the DNA of this book is emotional and psychological, whereas most diet books only think about the physical. If you can change you mind, you stand a better chance of improving the health of your body.

Many people believe that it takes extreme behaviors to improve your health, that you must completely redesign your life, and abandon all comfort. You've been led to believe that good health only exists on a path paved in discomfort. In an attempt to build resilience by abandoning comfort, you've embraced extremes that are designed to break you down rather than build you up. It's important to challenge your current way of life in order to improve your health. But, the journey looks nothing like the restriction-heavy, lifestyle-breaking plans you've been sold.

It's time to prioritize your mental and social health, and—in doing so—you'll improve your physical health. When you expand your comfort zone instead of abandoning it, you allow yourself to make gradual improvements and create habits that are built to survive the test of time and day-to-day stress. A stronger health foundation is established by keeping some of what you love and removing what does the most harm. And, no matter what, don't invest in the belief that there is no margin for error. That is the mistake most likely to break you physically, emotionally, and mentally. It's rarely the "imperfections" in our diets that cause the most damage—it's our overreactions to small decisions your body can handle. If the slingshot doesn't have enough tension, then you won't be sent spiraling.

That was the motivation for writing this book. You've been taught to judge every health behavior under a microscope, and the overanalysis is doing more harm than good. When trying to be healthy gets in the way of healthy living, enjoying social experiences, and feeling connected to your friends and your own body, that's when you know it's time to take a step back and reassess.

Believing you are healthy is the foundation of creating behaviors and habits that last. You must shift who you thought you were and embrace the person you can become. The thing that is holding you back is that negative, ultra-critical voice in your head.

Doing what works is more valuable than doing what's popular. It's why you need to find a way of living that truly works for you, even if it doesn't come with crazy claims or millions of social media likes. The best decision you can make is one that gets you off the hamster wheel of diets and trends and onto a direct path to the body you want.

Life is short. You should be happy, enjoy good food, and not let arguments about the best diet distract you from what really matters.

The goal of this book was not to encourage you to eat more takeout food. It was to stop you from thinking you couldn't live in the current food environment and still be healthy. This is rarely the message, and it's time to change the narrative. Frustration and discomfort are meant to be teachers—not the goal. I think you've taken your bruises and experienced enough struggles. It's time for success.

Your mind and body have an almost unlimited capacity to adjust, evolve, and improve—if you're in an environment that helps you thrive. Children don't learn in threatening environments. They grow with reinforcement and support. They don't start on their first day of math learning calculus. They start with the basic addition and subtraction and then progress. If you want to improve your endurance, you don't start by running ten miles on the first day. Sure, it causes pain and discomfort, but what do you gain? It's too much, too soon.

It's far more effective to build step-by-step, mile-by-mile, until ten miles feels like the first steps. And that was the point of this book. To provide a more effective way to go from zero to one—without always falling and starting back at zero—and then be able to easily springboard your way from one up to ten.

It's time to end the belief that better health requires constant suffering. Good changes reduce pain. Bad changes keep you in it. Optimal health is about understanding that your behaviors can be less than perfect and still be perfectly healthy.

As you start to play a new game, remember to leverage helpful tools instead of stressing overwhelming rules. Because now you understand what it takes to live a healthier life and how to stay on track in any situation.

And—no matter what life throws your way—be confident in your decisions and feel in control of your body because you know you can't screw this up.

ACKNOWLEDGMENTS

"People and experiences."

That's my answer when people ask me what I value most in life. And it's also what allowed me to write this book after so many years trying to figure out how to put this message on paper. If it weren't for many eye-opening experiences, and so many incredible, inspiring people, this book wouldn't be possible. And that includes the five hundred people who went on this journey with me and provided invaluable feedback that improved the program and clarified the lessons shared.

Even though this is my tenth book, it's my first solo, non-ghost-written project in nearly a decade. The project wouldn't be possible without my agents, Scott Hoffman and Steve Troha, and the publishing team at William Morrow. Your faith in me means the world, and I'm grateful that you supported my vision to write a health book that looked nothing like most other diet books. Thank you, in particular, to Cassie Jones and Jill Zimmerman for the endless work they put in making this book what it is today.

I don't think it's possible to thank everyone who matters, but I'd like to thank a few people in particular. To my Pen Name and Born Fitness teams, thank you for all your support.

Jordan Bornstein: You're my best friend and the best hire I ever made. Thanks for hanging with me as I endlessly dream big dreams. You continue to help me level up (and stop me from being my own worst enemy . . . sometimes). Kiki Garthwaite: You're a legend. Thank you for bringing to life all the beautiful illustrations that add the new dimension I've always wanted in a book.

BJ Ward and Natalie Sabin: I learn so much by watching you both coach our clients, and their stories are endless inspiration. Thank you for making the Born Fitness coaching experience what it is.

Special thanks to all the people who gave me their time to help me understand this incredibly complex topic. This includes Danielle Belardo, Dr. Stephan Guyenet, Dr. Spencer Nadolsky, Tamar Haspel, Dr. Nicola Guess, and Dr. Robert Kushner.

Much respect to those that have influenced me over the years and helped make the wellness space a better place. It's impossible to list everyone, but much appreciation to Dr. Andy Galpin, Dr. Layne Norton, Ben Bruno, and Luka Hocevar, to name a few.

Alan Aragon: You were the first person who helped me understand the possibility of pragmatic healthy eating. You are in a class of your own in the world of nutrition.

To James Clear and Ryan Holiday, thank you for creating books that helped me see a better path forward for wellness, and for taking the time to read some of this book to ensure I applied your ideas accurately. Mark Mason: Your ability to get to the heart of what matters has been groundbreaking for so many.

Tim Ferriss: Working with you changed the way I see the world and helped me ask questions that result in better solutions.

Jason Feifer: You've helped me level up for years. And without knowing it, you did it again.

Daniel Ketchell: You've supported me every step of the way, and I know we're still just getting started making the world a healthier place.

David Forsberg, Jen Widerstrom, Ben Lyons, Jonathan Yarmeisch, Patrick Noland, Naomi Piercey, and Neema Yazdani: You all know what you mean to me, and your support and friendship make these things possible. Olivia Langdon: Thanks for teaching me how to make healthy food taste delicious.

Ted Spiker: I'm not here without you. Thank you.

Kenzie Cozart: Thanks for being a part of our family and helping with the boys until I finished the manuscript.

Michael Easter: Thank you for reading, sharing your thoughts, and challenging me to share my message (and for your book, The Comfort Crisis).

Jack Gray, Kendall Selverian, Alex Braunschek, and Tori Rafanelli: My OG Ladder crew. Our journey helped me see what I needed to write. What a ride.

Mel, this is the "magic pill" you always asked me to create. I hope it honors your memory. Faye: thanks for raising my favorite human.

Cindy Crawford: I hope the whole world can follow your mentality and find happiness and health. Thank you for contributing to this project.

Arnold Schwarzenegger: You gave me the chance of a lifetime more than ten years ago, and I continue to keep an underdog mentality in everything I do. Thank for continuing to put your faith in me and supporting my desire to continue the fitness crusade you started.

Mom and Dad: I love you both. You raised me to believe I can do anything, and that includes helping people with my words. I don't always get it right, but I hope I make you proud. And Dad, you truly were the heartbeat of this book.

My brothers Josh and Aaron, I love you both. Thanks for supporting my desire to do one hundred things at once.

My sons, Bode and Asher. You give me purpose, meaning, and joy every day. I have a lot of jobs, but none of them hold a candle to being your dad. Thanks for being patient with me when I had to write instead of play. I hope this book shows you that we all have the superpower to help others, even those we don't know. I love you both more than you'll ever know.

And finally, my Queen B, Rachie. I could write an entire book about you, and there still wouldn't be enough words to express my love and appreciation. Because of you, I truly understand the connection between the mental and the physical, and that perspective has made all the difference in helping people. There is no one in the world like you. You make me a better man, husband, and father. Sorry for taking three years to get the paint off the upstairs window. But like I told you, it would all work out. You are forever my #1, and I love you with all my heart.

UNIVERSAL CONVERSION CHART

OVEN TEMPERATURE EQUIVALENTS

250°F = 120°C
275°F = 135°C
300°F = 150°C
325°F = 160°C
350°F = 180°C
375°F = 190°C
400°F = 200°C
425°F = 220°C
450°F = 230°C
475°F = 240°C
500°F = 260°C

MEASUREMENT EQUIVALENTS

Measurements should always be level unless directed otherwise.

⅛ teaspoon = 0.5 mL
¼ teaspoon = 1 mL
½ teaspoon = 2 mL
1 teaspoon = 5 mL
1 tablespoon = 3 teaspoons = ½ fluid ounce = 15 mL
2 tablespoons = ⅛ cup = 1 fluid ounce = 30 mL
4 tablespoons = ¼ cup = 2 fluid ounces = 60 mL
5⅓ tablespoons = ⅓ cup = 3 fluid ounces = 80 mL
8 tablespoons = ½ cup = 4 fluid ounces = 120 mL
10⅔ tablespoons = ⅔ cup = 5 fluid ounces = 160 mL
12 tablespoons = ¾ cup = 6 fluid ounces = 180 mL
16 tablespoons = 1 cup = 8 fluid ounces = 240 mL

NOTES

Introduction: Hope

1. Rand, Kathryn, Michael Vallis, and Sara F.L. Kirk. "'It is not the diet; it is the mental part we need help with.' A multilevel analysis of psychological, emotional, and social well-being in obesity," *International Journal of Qualitative Studies in Health and Well-Being*, 12, no. 1 (December 2017): 1306421, doi: 10.10^{80}/17482631.2017.1306421

Chapter 1: So Easy It's Hard to Fail

1. Gardner, Benjamin, Phillippa Lally, Jane Wardle. "Making health habitual: the psychology of 'habit-formation' and general practice," *The British Journal of General Practice*, 605, no. 62 (December 2012): 664–6.

Chapter 2: The Diet Game Is Fixed

1. Yaemsiri, S., M. M. Slining, S. K. Agarwal. "Perceived weight status, overweight diagnosis, and weight control among US adults: The NHANES 2003–2008 Study," *The International Journal of Obesity*, 35, no. 8 (August 2011): 1063–70.
2. Hall, Kevin D., Scott Kahan. "Maintenance of Lost Weight and Long-Term Management of Obesity," *Medical Clinics of North America*, 102, no. 1 (January 2018): 183–197.
3. Colombarolli, Maíra, Stivaleti Jônatas de Oliveira, Táki Athanássios Cordás. "Craving for carbs: food craving and disordered eating in low-carb dieters and its association with intermittent fasting," *Eating and Weight Disorders*, 23, no. 9 (August 2022): 1–9.
4. Dulloo, A. G., J. Jacquet, J.-P. Montani, Y. Schutz. "How dieting makes the lean fatter: from a perspective of body composition autoregulation through adipostats and protein-stats awaiting discovery," *Obesity Reviews*, 16, supplement 1 (February 2015): 25–35.
5. Tomiyama, A. Janet, Britt Ahlstrom, Traci Mann. "Long-term Effects of Dieting: Is Weight Loss Related to Health?" *Social and Personality Psychology Compass*, 7, no. 12 (December 2013): 861–877.
6. Ayyad, Carlos, Therese Andersen. "Long-term efficacy of dietary treatment of obesity: a systematic review of studies published between 1931 and 1999," *Obesity Reviews*, 2, no. 1 (December 2001): 113–119.
7. Soetens, Barbara, Caroline Braet, Leen Van Vlierberghe, Arne Roets. "Resisting temptation: effects of exposure to a forbidden food on eating behaviour," *Appetite*, 51, no. 1 (July 2008): 202–205.

Chapter 3: This Changes Everything

1. Duarte, Cristiana, Marcela Matos, R. James Stubbs, Corinne Gale, Liam Morris, Jose Pinto Gouveia, and Paul Gilbert. "The Impact of Shame, Self-Criticism and Social Rank on Eating Behaviours in Overweight and Obese Women Participating in a Weight Management Programme," *PLoS One*, 12, no. 1 (January 2017): https://doi.org/10.1371/journal.pone.0167571.

Chapter 4: The Paradox of Comfort

1. Alan S. Waterman. "When Effort Is Enjoyed: Two Studies of Intrinsic Motivation for Personally Salient Activities," *Motivation and Emotion*, 29, no. 9 (September 2005): 165–188.

Chapter 5: Seek Solutions, Not Scapegoats

1. Hall, Kevin D., I. Sadaf Farooqi, Jeffery M. Friedman, Samuel Klein, Ruth J. F. Loos, David J. Mangelsdorf, Stephen O'Rahilly, et. al. "The energy balance model of obesity: beyond calories in, calories out," *The American Journal of Clinical Nutrition,* 115, no. 5 (May 2022): 1243–1254.

2. Dansinger, Michael L., Joi Augustin Gleason, John L. Griffith, Harry P. Selker, Ernst J. Schaefer. "Comparison of the Atkins, Ornish, Weight Watchers, and Zone diets for weight loss and heart disease risk reduction: a randomized trial," *Journal of the American Medical Association,* 293, no. 1 (January 2005): 43–53.

3. Alhassan, S., S. Kim, A. Bersamin, A. C. King, C. D. Gardner. "Dietary adherence and weight loss success among overweight women: results from the A TO Z weight loss study," *International Journal of Obesity,* 32, no. 6 (June 2008): 985–991.

4. Hu, Tian, Katherine T. Mills, Lu Yao, Kathryn Demanelis, Mohamed Eloustaz, William S. Yancy Jr., Tanika N. Kelly, Jiang He, Lydia A. Bazzano, et al. "Effects of low-carbohydrate diets versus low-fat diets on metabolic risk factors: a meta-analysis of randomized controlled clinical trials," *American Journal of Epidemiology,* 176, supplement 7, (October 2012): S44-S54.

5. Bunzeck, Nico, Emrah Düzel. "Absolute coding of stimulus novelty in the human substantia nigra/VTA," *Neuron,* 51, no. 3 (August 2006): 369–379.

6. Ibid.

7. Del Corral, Pedro, David R. Bryan, W. Timothy Garvey, Barbara A. Gower, Gary R. Hunter. "Dietary adherence during weight loss predicts weight regain," *Obesity,* 19, no. 6 (June 2011): 1177–1181.

Chapter 6: Note from Your Future Self

1. Tomiyama, A. Janet, Traci Mann, and Shelley E. Taylor. "Low Calorie Dieting Increases Cortisol," *Psychosomatic Medicine,* 72, no. 4 (May 2010): 357–364.

2. Stacey R. Finkelstein, Ayelet Fishbach. "When Healthy Food Makes You Hungry," *Journal of Consumer Research,* Volume 37, Issue 3, October 2010, 357–367, https://doi.org/10.1086/652248

3. Bradley P Turnwald, J Parker Goyer, Danielle Z Boles, Amy Silder, Scott L Delp, Alia J Crum. "Learning one's genetic risk changes physiology independent of actual genetic risk," *Nature Human Behaviour,* 2019 Jan 3(1):48-56. doi: 10.1038/s41562-018-0483-4

4. Byrne, S., Z. Cooper, C. Fairburn. "Weight maintenance and relapse in obesity: a qualitative study," *International Journal of Obesity and Related Metabolic Disorders,* 27, no. 8 (August 2003): 955–962.

Chapter 7: The Trap Doors

1. Steele, Eurídice Martínez, Larissa Galastri Baraldi, and Carlos Augusto Monteiro. "Ultra-processed foods and added sugars in the US diet: evidence from a nationally representative cross-sectional study," *British Medical Journal,* 6, no. 3 (January 2016): e009892, doi: 10.1136/bmjopen-2015–009892.

2. Steele, Eurídice Martínez, Larissa Galastri Baraldi, and Carlos Augusto Monteiro. "Ultra-processed foods and added sugars in the US diet: evidence from a nationally representative cross-sectional study," *British Medical Journal,* 6, no. 3 (January 2016): e009892, doi: 10.1136/bmjopen-2015–009892.

3. Mathers, John C., Katherine M. Livingstone, Carlos Celis-Morales, George D. Papandonatos, Bahar Erar, Jose C. Florez, Kathleen A. Jablonski, Cristina Razquin. "FTO genotype and weight loss: systematic review and meta-analysis of 9563 individual participant data from eight randomised controlled trials," *British Medical Journal,* 354, i4707 (September 2016): https://doi.org/10.1136/bmj.i4707.

4. Pontzer, Herman, Yosuke Yamada, Hiroyuki Sagayama, Philip N. Ainslie, Lene F. Andersen, Liam J. Anderson Lenore Arab, et al. "Daily energy expenditure through the human life course," 373, no. 6556 (August 2021): 808–812.
5. Hall, Kevin D., Erin Fothergill, Juen Guo, Lilian Howard, Jennifer C. Kerns, Nicolas D. Knuth, Robert Brychta, et al. "Persistent metabolic adaptation 6 years after *The Biggest Loser* competition," *Obesity*, 24, no. 8 (August 2016): 1612–1619.

Chapter 8: I Will Teach You to Eat

1. Wong, Kapo, Alan H. S. Chan, and S. C. Ngan. "The Effect of Long Working Hours and Overtime on Occupational Health: A Meta-Analysis of Evidence from 1998 to 2018," *International Journal of Environmental Research and Public Health*, 16, no. 12 (June 2019): 2102, doi: 10.3390/ijerph16122102.
2. Antoni, Rona, Tracey M. Robertson, M. Denise Robertson, and Jonathan D. Johnston. "A pilot feasibility study exploring the effects of a moderate time-restricted feeding intervention on energy intake, adiposity and metabolic physiology in free-living human subjects," *Journal of Nutritional Science*, 22, no. 7 (July 2018): 1–6.
3. Gill, Shubhroz, Satchidananda Panda. "A Smartphone App Reveals Erratic Diurnal Eating Patterns in Humans that Can Be Modulated for Health Benefits," *Cell Metabolism*, 22, no. 5 (November 2015): 789–798.
4. Jakubowicz, Daniela, Julio Wainstein, Bo Ahren, Zohar Landau, Yosefa Bar-Dayan, Oren Froy. "Fasting until noon triggers increased postprandial hyperglycemia and impaired insulin response after lunch and dinner in individuals with type 2 diabetes: a randomized clinical trial," *Diabetes Care*, 38, no. 10 (October 2015): 1820–1826.
5. Ledikwe, Jenny H., Heidi M. Blanck, Laura Kettel Khan, Mary K. Serdula, Jennifer D. Seymour, Beth C. Tohill, Barbara J. Rolls. "Dietary energy density is associated with energy intake and weight status in US adults," *American Journal of Clinical Nutrition*, 83, no. 6 (June 2006): 1362–1368.
6. Stubbs, R. J., C. G. Harbron, P. R. Murgatroyd, A. M. Prentice. "Covert manipulation of dietary fat and energy density: effect on substrate flux and food intake in men eating ad libitum," *American Journal of Clinical Nutrition*, 62, no. 2 (August 1995): 316–329.
7. Weigle, David S., Patricia A. Breen, Colleen C. Matthys, Holly S. Callahan, Kaatje E. Meeuws, Verna R. Burden, Jonathan Q. Purnell. "A high-protein diet induces sustained reductions in appetite, ad libitum caloric intake, and body weight despite compensatory changes in diurnal plasma leptin and ghrelin concentrations," *The American Journal of Clinical Nutrition*, 82, no. 1 (July 2005): 41–48.
8. Reynolds, Andrew, Jim Mann, John Cummings, Nicola Winter, Evelyn Mete, Lisa Te Morenga. "Carbohydrate quality and human health: a series of systematic reviews and meta-analyses," *The Lancet*, 393, no. 10170 (February 2019): 435–445.
9. Simpson, S. J., D. Raubenheimer. "Obesity: the protein leverage hypothesis," *Obesity Reviews*, 6, no. 2 (April 2005): 133–142.
10. Rolls, B. J., P. M. Van Duijvenvoorde, E. T. Rolls. "Pleasantness changes and food intake in a varied four-course meal," *Appetite*, 5, no. 4 (December 1984): 337–348.
11. Roe, Liane S., Jennifer S. Meengs, Leann L. Birch, Barbara J. Rolls. "Serving a variety of vegetables and fruit as a snack increased intake in preschool children," *The American Journal of Clinical Nutrition*, 98, no. 3 (September 2013): 693–699.
12. Kergoata, Sophie Miquel, Veronique Azais-Braesco, Britt Burton-Freeman, Marion M. Hetherington. "Effects of chewing on appetite, food intake and gut hormones: A systematic review and meta-analysis," *Physiology & Behavior*, 151, no. 1 (November 2015): 88–96.
13. Robinson, Eric, Paul Aveyard, Amanda Daley, Kate Jolly, Amanda Lewis, Deborah Lycett, Suzanne Higgs. "Eating attentively: a systematic review and meta-analysis of the

effect of food intake memory and awareness on eating," *The American Journal of Clinical Nutrition*, 97, no. 4 (April 2013): 728–742.

14. Andrade, Ana M., Daniel L. Kresge, Pedro J. Teixeira, Fátima Baptista, Kathleen J. Melanson. "Does eating slowly influence appetite and energy intake when water intake is controlled?" *The International Journal of Behavioral Nutrition and Physical Activity*, 21, no. 9 (November 2012): 135.

15. "Eating More; Enjoying Less," Pew Research Center, last modified April 19, 2006, https://www.pewresearch.org/social-trends/2006/04/19/eating-more-enjoying-less/.

16. Hebebrand, Johannes, Özgür Albayrak, Roger Adan, Jochen Antel, Carlos Dieguez, Johannes de Jong, et al. "'Eating addiction,' rather than 'food addiction,' better captures addictive-like eating behavior," *Neuroscience and Biobehavioral Reviews*, 47 (November 2014): 295–306.

17. Wansinka, Brian, Pierre Chandon. "Slim by design: Redirecting the accidental drivers of mindless overeating," *Journal of Consumer Psychology*, 24, no. 3 (July 2014): 413–431.

18. Baskin, Ernest, Margarita Gorlin, Zoë Chance, Nathan Novemsky, Ravi Dhar, Kim Huskey, Michelle Hatzis. "Proximity of snacks to beverages increases food consumption in the workplace: A field study," *Appetite*, 103 (August 2016): 244–248.

19. "Food Allergies," American College of Allergy, Asthma, and Immunology, last modified February 25, 2021, http://acaai.org/resources/connect/ask-allergist/can-i-develop-allergy-eating-too-much-food.

20. Sayon-Orea, Carmen, Miguel A. Martinez-Gonzalez, Maira Bes-Rastrollo. "Alcohol consumption and body weight: a systematic review," *Nutrition Reviews*, 69, no. 8 (August 2011): 419–431. Crouse, J. R., S. M. Grundy. "Effects of alcohol on plasma lipoproteins and cholesterol and triglyceride metabolism in man," *Journal of Lipid Research*, 25, no. 5 (May 1984): 486–496.

21. Cederbaum, Arthur. "Alcohol Metabolism," *Clinics in Liver Disease*, 16, no. 4 (November 2012): 667–685.

22. Traversy, Gregory, and Jean-Philippe Chaput. "Alcohol Consumption and Obesity: An Update," *Current Obesity Reports*, 4, no. 1 (March 2015): 122–130.

23. Schütze, M., M. Schulz, A. Steffen, M. M. Bergmann, A. Kroke, L. Lissner, H. Boeing. "Beer consumption and the 'beer belly': scientific basis or common belief?" *European Journal of Clinical Nutrition*, 63, no. 9 (September 2009): 1143–1149.

24. O'Keefe, James H., Salman K. Bhatti, Ata Bajwa, James J. DiNicolantonio, Carl J. Lavie. "Alcohol and cardiovascular health: the dose makes the poison . . . or the remedy," Mayo Clinic Proceedings, 89, no. 3 (March 2014): 382–393.

25. Yeomans, Martin R. "Alcohol, appetite and energy balance: is alcohol intake a risk factor for obesity?" *Physiology & Behavior*, 100, no. 1 (April 2010): 82–89.

Chapter 9: Let's Order Takeout

1. Todd, Jessica E., Lisa Mancino, and Biing-Hwan Lin. "The Impact of Food Away From Home on Adult Diet Quality," USDA Economic Research Report, 90 (February 2010): 1–24.

2. Urban, Lorien E., Alice H. Lichtenstein, Christine E .Gary, Jamie L. Fierstein, Ashley Equi, Carolyn Kussmaul, Gerard E. Dallal, et al. "The energy content of restaurant foods without stated calorie information," *Journal of the American Medical Association*, 173, no. 14 (July 2013): 1292–1299.

Chapter 12: The Plan That Never Stops Working

1. Byrne, N. M., A. Sainsbury, N. A. King, A. P. Hills, R. E. Wood. "Intermittent energy restriction improves weight loss efficiency in obese men: the MATADOR study," *International Journal of Obesity*, 42, no. 2 (February 2018): 129–138.

2. Nedeltcheva, Arlet V., Jennifer M. Kilkus, Jacqueline Imperial, Dale A. Schoeller, Plamen D. Penev. "Insufficient sleep undermines dietary efforts to reduce adiposity," *Annals of Internal Medicine,* 153, no. 7 (October 2010): 435–441.

3. Broussard, Josiane L., David A. Ehrmann, Eve Van Cauter, Esra Tasali, Matthew J. Brady. "Impaired insulin signaling in human adipocytes after experimental sleep restriction: a randomized, crossover study," *Annals of Internal Medicine,* 157, no. 8 (October 2012): 549–557.

4. Mosavat, Maryam, Mitra Mirsanjari, Diana Arabiat, Aisling Smyth, Lisa Whitehead. "The Role of Sleep Curtailment on Leptin Levels in Obesity and Diabetes Mellitus," *Obesity Fact,* 14, no. 2 (March 2021): 214–221.

5. Taheri, Shahrad, Ling Lin, Diane Austin, Terry Young, Emmanuel Mignot. "Short sleep duration is associated with reduced leptin, elevated ghrelin, and increased body mass index," *PLoS Medicine,* 3, no. 62 (December 2004): e62.

6. Greer, Stephanie M., Andrea N. Goldstein, Matthew P. Walker. "The impact of sleep deprivation on food desire in the human brain," *Nature Communications,* 4, 2259 (August 2013): doi: 10.1038/ncomms3259.

7. Hogenkamp, Pleunie S., Emil Nilsson, Victor C. Nilsson, Colin D. Chapman, Heike Vogel, Lina S. Lundberg, Sanaz Zarei, et al. "Acute sleep deprivation increases portion size and affects food choice in young men," *Psychoneuroendocrinology,* 38, no. 9 (February 2013): 1668–1674.

8. Drake, Christopher, Timothy Roehrs, John Shambroom, Thomas Roth. "Caffeine effects on sleep taken 0, 3, or 6 hours before going to bed," *Journal of Clinical Sleep Medicine,* 9, no. 11 (November 2013): 1195–1200.

9. Ibid.

10. McHill, Andrew W., Benjamin J. Smith, Kenneth P. Wright Jr. "Effects of caffeine on skin and core temperatures, alertness, and recovery sleep during circadian misalignment," *Journal of Biological Rhythms,* 29, no. 2 (April 2014): 131–143.

11. Scullin, Michael K., Madison L. Krueger, Hannah K. Ballard, Natalya Pruett, Donald L. Bliwise. "The effects of bedtime writing on difficulty falling asleep: A polysomnographic study comparing to-do lists and completed activity lists," *Journal of Experimental Psychology,* 147, no. 1 (January 2018): 139–146.

Chapter 13: Putting It All Together

1. Dallosso, H. M., P. R. Murgatroyd, W. P. James. "Feeding frequency and energy balance in adult males," *Human Nutrition Clinical Nutrition,* 36C, no. 1 (1982): 25–39.

    W P Verboeket-van de Venne, K R Westerterp, "Influence of the feeding frequency on nutrient utilization in man: consequences for energy metabolism," European Journal of Clinical Nutrition, 45, no. 3, (March 1991): 161–169.

    Verboeket-van de Venne, W. P., K. R. Westerterp. "Frequency of feeding, weight reduction and energy metabolism," *International Journal of Obesity and Other Related Metabolic Disorders,* 17, no. 1 (January 1993): 31–36.

    Verboeket-van de Venne, W. P., K. R. Westerterp, A. D. Kester. "Effect of the pattern of food intake on human energy metabolism," *British Journal of Nutrition,* 70, no. 1 (July 1993): 103–115.

    Smeets, Astrid J., Margriet S. Westerterp-Plantenga. "Acute effects on metabolism and appetite profile of one meal difference in the lower range of meal frequency," *British Journal of Nutrition,* 99, no. 6 (June 2008): 1316–1321.

2. Higgins, Kelly A., Joshua L. Hudson, Anna M. R. Hayes, Ethan Braun, Eunjin Cheon, Sam C. Couture, Nilupa S. Gunaratna. "Systematic Review and Meta-Analysis on the Effect of Portion Size and Ingestive Frequency on Energy Intake and Body Weight among Adults in Randomized Controlled Feeding Trials," *Advances in Nutrition,* 13, no. 1 (February 2022): 248–268.

3. Murakami, Kentaro M., Barbara E. Livingstone, Hitomi Okubo, Satoshi Sasaki. "Prevalence and characteristics of misreporting of energy intake in Japanese adults: the 2012 National Health and Nutrition Survey," *Asian Pacific Journal of Clinical Nutrition,* 27, no. 2 (2018): 441–450.

Chapter 14: Movement Medicine: The 6-Week Plan

1. Pontzer, Herman, Ramon Durazo Arvizu, Lara R. Dugas, Jacob Plange Rhule, Pascal Bovet, Terrence E. Forrester, Estelle V. Lambert. "Constrained Total Energy Expenditure and Metabolic Adaptation to Physical Activity in Adult Humans," *Current Biology,* 26, no. 3 (February 2016): 410–417.
2. Thurber, Caitlin, Lara R. Dugas, Cara Ocobock, Bryce Carlson, John R. Speakman, Herman Pontzer. "Extreme events reveal an alimentary limit on sustained maximal human energy expenditure," *Science Advances,* 5, no. 6 (June 2019): eaaw0341.

INDEX

ABOUT THE AUTHOR

ADAM BORNSTEIN is a *New York Times* bestselling author and an award-winning writer and editor. He is the founder of Born Fitness and Pen Name Consulting and a cofounder of The Pump. Previously, he was the chief nutrition officer at Ladder, the fitness and nutrition editor for *Men's Health*, the editorial director at LIVESTRONG.com, and a columnist for *Entrepreneur, Shape, Men's Fitness*, and *Muscle & Fitness*. He's authored or coauthored six books and has ghostwritten three other bestselling advice books. Bornstein is a nutrition adviser for many entrepreneurs, celebrities, and athletes, including LeBron James, Cindy Crawford, and Arnold Schwarzenegger. He lives in Denver with his wife and two sons.